HEALTH CARE IN TRANSITION

PATIENT SATISFACTION

DETERMINANTS, PSYCHOLOGICAL IMPLICATIONS AND IMPACT ON QUALITY OF LIFE

HEALTH CARE IN TRANSITION

Additional books and e-books in this series can be found
on Nova's website under the Series tab.

HEALTH CARE IN TRANSITION

PATIENT SATISFACTION

DETERMINANTS, PSYCHOLOGICAL IMPLICATIONS AND IMPACT ON QUALITY OF LIFE

DIELLE MORNEAU
EDITOR

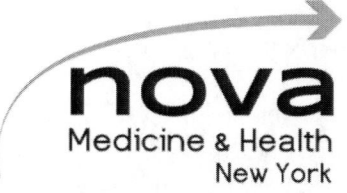

Copyright © 2020 by Nova Science Publishers, Inc.

All rights reserved. No part of this book may be reproduced, stored in a retrieval system or transmitted in any form or by any means: electronic, electrostatic, magnetic, tape, mechanical photocopying, recording or otherwise without the written permission of the Publisher.

We have partnered with Copyright Clearance Center to make it easy for you to obtain permissions to reuse content from this publication. Simply navigate to this publication's page on Nova's website and locate the "Get Permission" button below the title description. This button is linked directly to the title's permission page on copyright.com. Alternatively, you can visit copyright.com and search by title, ISBN, or ISSN.

For further questions about using the service on copyright.com, please contact:
Copyright Clearance Center
Phone: +1-(978) 750-8400　　　　Fax: +1-(978) 750-4470　　　　E-mail: info@copyright.com.

NOTICE TO THE READER

The Publisher has taken reasonable care in the preparation of this book, but makes no expressed or implied warranty of any kind and assumes no responsibility for any errors or omissions. No liability is assumed for incidental or consequential damages in connection with or arising out of information contained in this book. The Publisher shall not be liable for any special, consequential, or exemplary damages resulting, in whole or in part, from the readers' use of, or reliance upon, this material. Any parts of this book based on government reports are so indicated and copyright is claimed for those parts to the extent applicable to compilations of such works.

Independent verification should be sought for any data, advice or recommendations contained in this book. In addition, no responsibility is assumed by the Publisher for any injury and/or damage to persons or property arising from any methods, products, instructions, ideas or otherwise contained in this publication.

This publication is designed to provide accurate and authoritative information with regard to the subject matter covered herein. It is sold with the clear understanding that the Publisher is not engaged in rendering legal or any other professional services. If legal or any other expert assistance is required, the services of a competent person should be sought. FROM A DECLARATION OF PARTICIPANTS JOINTLY ADOPTED BY A COMMITTEE OF THE AMERICAN BAR ASSOCIATION AND A COMMITTEE OF PUBLISHERS.

Additional color graphics may be available in the e-book version of this book.

Library of Congress Cataloging-in-Publication Data

Names: Morneau, Dielle, editor. Title: Patient satisfaction: : determinants, psychological implications and impact on quality of life / Dielle Morneau. Description: Hauppauge : Nova Science Publishers, 2020. | Series: Health care in transition | Includes bibliographical references and index. | Summary: "Patient Satisfaction: Determinants, Psychological Implications and Impact on Quality of Life first provides an in-depth, evidence-based review of the patient outcomes associated with patient experience measures across a wide range of specialties and settings. The authors describe the instruments used to assess patient and family satisfaction, focusing on the presentation of various factors related to satisfaction in the field of child and adolescent psychiatry. Current literature on the factors which impact patient quality of life are explored and reviewed in the context of breast reconstruction, using assessment tools such as the BREAST-Q"--Provided by publisher. Identifiers: LCCN 2020039703 (print) | LCCN 2020039704 (ebook) |
ISBN 9781536186130 (paperback) | ISBN 9781536186390 (adobe pdf)
Classification: LCC R727.3 (print) | LCC R727.3 (ebook) | DDC 362.1--dc23
LC record available at https://lccn.loc.gov/2020039703
LC ebook record available at https://lccn.loc.gov/2020039704

Published by Nova Science Publishers, Inc. † New York

CONTENTS

Preface		vii
Chapter 1	Outcomes Associated with Patient Experience Measures *Joshua J. Davis*	1
Chapter 2	Satisfaction within Child and Adolescent Mental Health Service from Multiple Perspectives *Marina Gouhaut, Carole Kapp, Hélène Beutler, Kerstin Jessica von Plessen and Sébastien Urben*	67
Chapter 3	Breast Reconstruction: A Review of Factors Affecting Patient Satisfaction and Quality of Life *Maleka Ramji and Farrah Yau*	99
Index		121

PREFACE

Patient Satisfaction: Determinants, Psychological Implications and Impact on Quality of Life first provides an in-depth, evidence-based review of the patient outcomes associated with patient experience measures across a wide range of specialties and settings.

The authors describe the instruments used to assess patient and family satisfaction, focusing on the presentation of various factors related to satisfaction in the field of child and adolescent psychiatry.

Current literature on the factors which impact patient quality of life are explored and reviewed in the context of breast reconstruction, using assessment tools such as the BREAST-Q.

Chapter 1 - Recent changes in healthcare models over the last 2 decades have led to an increased focus on patient experience and satisfaction measures. Given improved experience has an inherent value to patients and families, patient experience is arguably a valid standalone outcome. These measures are now tied to reimbursement, as well. Importantly, though, patient experience must be tied to improved or, at least, not worsened patient outcomes to make sure this measure is appropriately emphasized. Many healthcare providers opine about an over-emphasis on patient satisfaction leading to unnecessary medical tests and treatments. Others, though, would argue that adequate communication between physicians and patients can abate this perceived need to "do" more. Patient satisfaction has been associated with improved medication adherence in the outpatient setting and improved long-term outcomes after hospitalization. However, other studies have shown higher satisfaction associated with increased healthcare use and increased mortality. This chapter will take an in-depth evidence-based review of the evidence on patient outcomes associated with patient experience measures across a wide range of specialties and settings.

Chapter 2 - Within the context of Child and Adolescent Mental Health Service (CAMHS), patient's and families' satisfaction is of great importance in psychotherapeutic treatment because it is closely linked to positive clinical improvements as well as to subsequent requests for help. Furthermore, the integration of multiple perspectives (e.g., children/adolescents, parents, clinicians) is of crucial importance. Therefore, in this chapter the authors will, first, describe the instruments used to assess satisfaction. Afterwards, the authors will focus on the presentation of the various factors related to satisfaction in the field of child and adolescent psychiatry. In particular, the authors will focus on the determinants such as the intra-individual characteristics, the inter-personal dimensions, treatment outcomes, the organization of care/services and the expectations. More specifically, the authors will describe these factors from different perspectives (i.e., children/adolescents, parents, clinicians) and in different types of treatment (i.e., out- and inpatient). The last part of the chapter will be devoted to identifying the limits in identifying satisfaction determinants and proposing avenues for future researches. The chapter is enriched by clinical examples to illustrate the described theoretical aspects.

Chapter 3 - Breast cancer is the most common cancer affecting women worldwide, with one in eight females diagnosed before the age of 85 years. Many survivors are young and live on for decades following treatment with 5-year survival rates as high as 90%. Oncologic management of breast cancer includes lumpectomy with adjuvant radiation or mastectomy alone. This choice is impacted by a myriad of factors, relying on a shared decision-making process between the breast surgeon and patient. Over the years, the authors have seen an increasing trend for mastectomy, which often has a significant impact on a woman's quality of life, body image and sexuality. For decades, breast reconstruction, both autologous and alloplastic has been relied upon to address these concerns and impart a sense of 'wholeness' for women. Reconstruction also allows women to limit their use of external prosthesis and wear a greater variety of clothing. There are many factors that impact patient satisfaction and quality of life, following breast reconstruction. This chapter will explore and review current literature on what these factors are and their impact on patient quality of life. With health-related quality of life (HRQoL) central to the success of breast reconstruction, the study and measurement of patient reported outcomes (PROs) has allowed surgeons to evaluate these factors with greater thoughtfulness. Assessment tools such as the BREAST-Q have been designed for evaluating outcomes in breast reconstruction and remains the most frequently used validated breast reconstructive questionnaire. Several surgical factors have been identified as being key players impacting patient reported outcomes. These include the type of reconstruction performed (autologous versus alloplastic and the type of implant used), the timing of the reconstruction and whether surgery is unilateral or bilateral. Additional factors have also been distilled that have received increased attention in recent years. These include clinical variables, psychosocial variables and sociodemographic variables. Understanding these factors is vitally important for surgeons performing breast reconstructive procedures, to enhance quality of care, address patient's expectations and optimize future breast surgery research.

In: Patient Satisfaction
Editor: Dielle Morneau

ISBN: 978-1-53618-613-0
© 2020 Nova Science Publishers, Inc.

Chapter 1

OUTCOMES ASSOCIATED WITH PATIENT EXPERIENCE MEASURES

Joshua J. Davis[*], *MD*
Vituity, Wichita, KS, US

ABSTRACT

Recent changes in healthcare models over the last 2 decades have led to an increased focus on patient experience and satisfaction measures. Given improved experience has an inherent value to patients and families, patient experience is arguably a valid standalone outcome. These measures are now tied to reimbursement, as well. Importantly, though, patient experience must be tied to improved or, at least, not worsened patient outcomes to make sure this measure is appropriately emphasized.

Many healthcare providers opine about an over-emphasis on patient satisfaction leading to unnecessary medical tests and treatments. Others, though, would argue that adequate communication between physicians and patients can abate this perceived need to "do" more.

Patient satisfaction has been associated with improved medication adherence in the outpatient setting and improved long-term outcomes after hospitalization. However, other studies have shown higher

---

[*] Corresponding Author's E-mail: jjvwd@udel.edu.

satisfaction associated with increased healthcare use and increased mortality. This chapter will take an in-depth evidence-based review of the evidence on patient outcomes associated with patient experience measures across a wide range of specialties and settings.

INTRODUCTION

Since the early 2000s, an increased focus has been placed on measuring patient's perceptions of their own care, i.e., patient experience or patient satisfaction. Patient satisfaction and patient experience are closely related constructs. Patient satisfaction is a subjective measure about whether a patient's expectations regarding their care were met (Agency for Healthcare Research and Quality 2017). Patient experience, on the other hand, is a construct that encompasses the patient's perceptions of their interactions with the health care system. Patient satisfaction is quite easy to measure. However, patient experience has historically been difficult to measure due to its lack of definition and quantifiability. One prominent definition from leading healthcare consulting firm The Beryl Institute is "the sum of all interactions, shaped by an organization's culture, that influence patient perceptions across the continuum of care" (The Beryl Institute 2020). Several tools exist that attempt to measure and quantify patient experience (Beattie et al. 2015), which include HCAHPS, the Press-Ganey® proprietary survey (Press Ganey 2020), Quality from the Patient's Perspective (Wilde et al. 1994), and the Patient Satisfaction Questionnaire (now in its third version) (RAND 2020; Ware, Davies-Avery, and Stewart 1978). The most robust evidence for these tools is for the inpatient setting, but tools for the emergency department (Male et al. 2020) and outpatient care (Saila et al. 2008) have also been developed. Despite difficulties in measuring patient experience, most healthcare organizations recognize that it is an important aspect of high-quality and patient-centered care (Agency for Healthcare Research and Quality 2017).

The focus on patient experience was spurred by the Institute of Medicine's landmark publication *Crossing the Quality Chasm* in 2001 and the subsequent development and use of the Hospital Consumer Assessment of Healthcare Providers and Systems (HCAHPS) by the Center for Medicare and Medicaid Services (CMS) and the Agency for Healthcare Research and Quality (AHRQ) (2020). In 2007, collection and public reporting of patient satisfaction data through HCAHPS became tied to reimbursement for hospitals, and in 2012, patient satisfaction values were tied to value-based reimbursement incentives. Thus, hospitals have a financial incentive to improve patient satisfaction.

Besides financial incentives, there are several reasons why patient experience should be measured. Many prominent leaders in the field (Berwick 2009) and national organizations from several countries (Agency for Healthcare Research and Quality 2017; Australian Commission on Safety and Quality in Health Care 2012; Fujisawa and Klazinga 2017; National Institute for Health and Care Excellence 2012) would argue that patient experience is a quality measure in itself. Further, measurement of patient experience allows consumers to compare aspects of healthcare that are not measured reliably elsewhere. Patients, too, can offer insight and unique perspectives into quality issues and potential solutions.

However, many clinicians argue that patients may not know what is in their best interest and may not be able to accurately evaluate healthcare quality. To these clinicians, patient experience must be tied to beneficial outcomes beyond the measure of experience itself. Patient satisfaction has been tied to many beneficial outcomes (Cathal, Lennox, and Bell 2013; Stewart 1995); however, one of the most controversial studies in patient experience, "The Cost of Satisfaction," showed that higher patient satisfaction was associated with increased mortality (Fenton et al. 2012). Therefore, the role of patient experience measures was further thrown into question. This chapter explores the evidence of how patient experience is tied to other healthcare quality outcomes.

GENERAL OUTPATIENT PRIMARY CARE

There are over 800 million outpatient visits (Centers for Disease control and Prevention 2020) in the United States each year, and as of

2018, revenue from outpatient care is nearly equal to that of inpatient care (American Hospital Association 2020). Outpatient care is a unique environment where patients have more choices regarding their care and care relationships are longitudinal. This provides unique drivers of patient experience compared to other settings. Most studies in outpatient care focus on a provider's role in the patient's experience (i.e., communication, collaboration, continuity, etc.) rather than systemic or practice issues (i.e., wait times, parking, etc.). Further, most research is on specific domains of patient experience or patient satisfaction and not using validated patient experience tools, i.e., Consumer Assessment of Healthcare Providers and Systems (CAHPS).

Mortality is perhaps the most important patient-related outcomes. One large, well-known study in 2012 showed an association with increased satisfaction and mortality (Fenton et al. 2012). A more recent study showed women were particularly at risk for mortality associated with increased satisfaction rates (Jerant et al. 2019).

It is not surprising that patient experience drives patient selection of physician practices and loyalty to physicians. For example, in Veterans with access to both Medicaid and Veteran's Affairs (VA) insurance, patient experience was shown to drive over 10% of patient's transitioning from VA services to Medicaid services (Wong et al. 2019). A study on over 17,000 patients showed that satisfaction with a visit predicted future attrition from providers (Rubin et al. 1993). In addition, Safran et al. (2001) showed that both personal and systemic aspects of patient experience drove patients voluntarily changing primary care physicians. Patient perceptions of their physician's knowledge, communication, and family-orientation are also known to be associated with older patients who voluntarily change doctors (Mold, Fryer, and Roberts 2004). Patient experience and satisfaction is also associated with loyalty in England, India, Iran, Taiwan, and Yemen (Anbori et al. 2010; Billinghurst and Whitfield 1993; Kondasani and Panda 2015; Nagraj et al. 2013; Rostami et al. 2019; Wang, Huang, and Howng 2011).

One of the most well-known associations of patient experience on outcomes is improved medication adherence. The relationship between patient-physician communication and adherence holds across specialties, ages, and chronicity of care (Arbuthnott and Sharpe 2009; Zolnierek and DiMatteo 2009). Medication adherence, though, is a surrogate, albeit important, outcome. That is, medication adherence is not patient-oriented itself, but is thought to be related to patient-oriented outcomes like mortality and hospitalization. However, it is important to acknowledge that not all surrogate outcomes do, in fact, relate to patient-oriented outcomes, despite intuition to the contrary (D'Agostino 2000).

Patient experience has been reliably shown to improve anti-hypertensive medication adherence (Fortuna et al. 2018; Schoenthaler et al. 2009). Notably, quantity of patient-physician time was not a predictor in one of these studies, suggesting quality of communication is a more important factor than quantity of physician time with patients (Fortuna et al. 2018). This is further evidenced by data on cancer screening showing that recommendation alone is not sufficient to improve adherence (Peterson et al. 2016). Another study looking at factors influencing medication adherence in patients with diabetes and high cholesterol showed physician communication, particularly at initial prescribing, was one of the major contributors to improved adherence (Molfenter and Brown 2014). A study in HIV patients showed that patient-provider interaction, but not patient satisfaction, was associated with improved medication adherence (Oetzel et al. 2015). Relationships between patient-physician communication and medication adherence carry over to asthma (Amin et al. 2020; Barnes and Ulrik 2015; Pelaez et al. 2015), cardiovascular disease (Okunrintemi et al. 2017), cancer screening (Peterson et al. 2016; Carcaise-Edinboro and Bradley 2008), diabetes (Bakar, Fahrini, and Kahn 2016; Nasir, Ariffin, and Yasin 2018; Schoenthaler et al. 2012), skin conditions (Hodari et al. 2006; Neri et al. 2019; Richards, Fortune, and Griffiths 2006; Thorneloe et al. 2013), stroke (Cheiloudaki and Alesopolous 2019; Kronish et al. 2013), and vaccination rates (Rao et al. 2006). Patients perceptions of doctor-patient relationship also affected reported medication adherence in 24 European countries, as well (Stavropoulou 2011). Importantly, physicians can be trained on communication techniques to improve adherence. A meta-analysis of 21 studies showed statistically improved odds of patient medication adherence with physician communication interventions (Zolnierek and Dimatteo 2009).

Older studies have shown improved patient-provider communication is also associated with a lower risk of malpractice in primary care (Levinson et al. 1997; Vincent 2003). Both sued physicians and the patients suing them agreed that improved doctor-patient communication was the most effective method to reduce malpractice claims (Shapiro et al. 1989). But more recent smaller studies have shown no association between patient experience measures and malpractice risk (Rodriguez et al. 2008), and that patients cannot accurately identify true medical errors (Solberg et al. 2008).

Improved communication and satisfaction can show reduced health care utilization, as well. In pediatric asthma, positive perception of physicians is associated with reduced emergency department visits and hospitalizations (Cabana et al. 2006; Clark et al. 2008). This is true in heart disease (Okunrintemi et al. 2017) and hepatobiliary disease, too (Cerier et al. 2018; Chen et al. 2018). Patients with a high perception of quality of their primary care and satisfaction are less likely to use the emergency department for nonemergent issues (Cowling, Majeed, and Harris 2018; Xin 2019). In the US, good patient experience is associated with decreased healthcare utilization and expenditures (Nasir and Okunrintemi 2019). In the United Kingdom (UK) and Canada, patient perceptions of their relationship with their doctor and patient centered-ness, respectively, are associated reduced number of referrals (Little et al. 2001; Stewart et al. 2000). However, one study showed that high baseline emergency department use was associated with low satisfaction, again highlighting difficulties with using retrospective studies to infer direction of correlation (or causation) (Chen et al. 2019). In addition, one large study showed increased satisfaction was associated with decreased emergency department use but increase inpatient use and higher overall health care expenditures (Fenton et al. 2012).

Access to care is another aspect of patient experience beyond satisfaction or communication. Increasing access to care could also reduce healthcare utilization. The benefits of having a primary care physician are diminished when patients have trouble with access to care (Rust et al. 2008). Poor access to care is associated with increased admissions for cancer (Bottle et al. 2012), diabetes (Calderon-Larranaga et al. 2014a), epilepsy (Calderon-Larranaga et al. 2014b), COPD (Calderon-Larranaga et al. 2011), pediatrics (Cecil et al. 2016), and stroke (Soljak et al. 2011). A large randomized trial of intensive primary care, though, showed increased readmission among VA patients with diabetes, chronic obstructive pulmonary disease, or congestive heart failure who received the intensive primary care intervention (Weinberger, Oddone, and Henderson 1996). Internationally, increased access to primary care is inconsistently associated with reduced emergency department use (Cowling et al. 2013; Harris, Patel, and Bowen 2011; Martin et al. 2002; O'Malley 2013; van den Berg, van Loenen, and Westert 2016; Whittaker et al. 2016), but the body of data on interventions designed to increase access is inconclusive (Ismail, Gibbons, and Gnani 2013).

Patient perceptions of care are associated with improved health status and health-related quality of life (QoL). In France, health-related QoL among those with addiction and dependence was associated with patient satisfaction (Muller et al. 2020). In India, parental reports of quality of care for their adolescents was associated with health-related QoL (Agnihotri and Awasthi 2012). In a Canadian study, both objective (video-taped) and patient-reported levels of patient-centered care are associated with improved self-reported health status (Stewart et al. 2000). In UK patients with cardiovascular disease, satisfaction was associated with symptoms and quality of life (Asadi-Lari, Packham, and Gray 2003). However, in the UK a study showed patient centered-ness was associated with patient satisfaction but not health status (Kinnersley et al. 1999). Increased patient health status is associated with increased patient satisfaction, though causation cannot be proven given the retrospective nature of studies (Ren et al. 2001; Xiao and Barber 2008). That is, patients with improved health status might report higher satisfaction at baseline and it may not be a result of their satisfaction/experience.

In primary care, several specific disease processes have been studied. One of the most well-studied of these is diabetes. Improved experience is associated with lower glycosylated hemoglobin (A1c) (better controlled diabetes) (Cinar and Schou 2014; Greenfield et al. 1988; Lee and Lin 2010; Linetzky et al. 2017), including when using online ratings (Emmert et al. 2015); though, the association is not universal (Al Shahrani and Baraja 2014) and this, too, is a surrogate outcome. Patient's rating of provider communication is also associated with greater self-care in diabetes (Chen, Lee, and Kuo 2012; Heisler et al. 2002). Interestingly, providing guideline-appropriate care has been associated with increased patient satisfaction (Gross et al. 2003; Narayan et al. 2003) Overall, improved patient experience appears to be associated with improved surrogate outcomes in diabetes care.

Chronic pain is another well studied disease process in primary care. In a randomized trial of patients with chronic pain disorders, a patient-centered approach by physicians was associated with reduced pain and anxiety (Alamo, Moral, and Perula de Torres 2002; McCracken, Evon, and Karapas 2002). Patient satisfaction is also associated with decreased pain scores at 1 year in patients with low back pain (Henschke et al. 2013). However, patient satisfaction is also associated with increased opioid prescriptions (Jerant, Agnoli, and Franks 2020; Sites et al. 2018) and misuse of opioid prescriptions (Lewis, Combs, and Trafton 2010). But, in some retrospective analyses, reduced opioid use by chronic pain patients is not associated with resultant reductions in patient satisfaction (Gewandter et al. 2018; Sharp et al. 2018), In one private pain clinic, functional outcomes were not associated with satisfaction (Dragovich et al. 2017). There is mixed data on whether patient experience is associated with improved pain in chronic pain issues.

Patient experience is not always associated with other quality measures, though. Studies using health plan data showed no correlation between patient experience and other common quality measures (Schneider et al. 2001; Sequist et al. 2008). An analysis in England showed that patient experience is not reliably associated with other aspects of clinical quality or patient outcomes, suggesting that patient experience could be a standalone measure but not used as a proxy for other elements of quality (Llanwarne et al. 2013). Others have shown that patient's ratings of quality of care do not correlate with other objective assessments of quality (Chang et al. 2006; Rao et al. 2006).

Despite the positive associations, a focus on patient satisfaction can lead to over-testing and inappropriate treatment. For example, simulated patients exposed to direct to consumer depression advertisements were more likely to be prescribed brand specific medication (Kravitz et al. 2005). Physicians with compensation tied to satisfaction are more likely to pursue guideline discordant advanced imaging for low back pain (Pham et al. 2009) and provide increased prescriptions for opioids (Carrico et al. 2018). However, the relationship to satisfaction and opioids is not consistent in all studies (Nalliah et al. 2020; North et al. 2018). Patients who expected and did not receive an antibiotic for lower respiratory tract infection, despite whether their physician thought it was necessary, were more likely to express dissatisfaction and return to care (Macfarlane et al. 1997). In a randomized trial, patients who presented with chest pain were also more likely to rate their care better than usual if they received testing (Sox, Marguiles, and Sox 1981).

In summary, there is conflicting evidence for the association between improved aspects of patient experience in primary care and other quality outcomes. Most outcomes with positive associations are surrogate outcomes, with the strongest evidence for medication adherence and diabetes care. One large trial showed increased mortality and hospital use with increased satisfaction. There is also potential for increased harm associated with improving satisfaction, namely increased testing and treatments that are not indicated. This will be exacerbated if balancing measures to satisfaction are not employed. Most data on patient experience in outpatient primary care focuses on communication and few studies used validated global patient experience scores or tools. Further, data is largely observational and the role of interventions that increase patient experience to improve other health outcomes is extremely limited.

GENERAL INPATIENT CARE

Inpatient hospital care was the first location to have patient satisfaction tied to reimbursement. Therefore, this domain has had a large number of analyses completed. Overall inpatient satisfaction is associated with reduced 30-day readmissions (Boulding et al. 2011), and quality measures including: postoperative bleeding, venous thromboembolism, pneumonia, sepsis, nosocomial infections, and decubitus ulcers (Isaac et al. 2010; Johnston et al. 2016). It was also tied to improved outcomes in acute myocardial infarction, congestive heart failure, surgery, and pneumonia (Isaac et al. 2010; Jha et al. 2008). But, one study showed only certain aspects of the HCAHPS survey (nurses listening and doctors explain information) were associated with decreased readmissions, and doctors and nurses asking about help at home was surprisingly associated with increased readmissions (Hachem et al. 2014) and another study suggested that, while satisfaction is associated with decreased 30-day readmissions, it may be that that poor satisfaction is due to being readmitted and not because of it (Siddiqui et al. 2018). This, again, highlights the limitations of retrospective data.

Online ratings are another measure of satisfaction and are associated with lower readmissions (Glover et al. 2015) and decreased mortality overall (Timian et al. 2013) and specifically for myocardial infarction and pneumonia (Bardach et al. 2013). Online ratings were also associated patient reported quality and decreased 30-day mortality in Norway (Bjertnaes et al. 2020), but not in a sample in New York State (Campbell and Li 2018). Perez and Freedman (2018) showed that online ratings were associated with quality measures, whereas Chen, Revere, and Black (2017) showed mixed results of traditional satisfaction and quality measures between academic and non-academic institutions, but academic hospitals did have higher "likelihood to recommend" and lower mortality.

There are several other singular studies on individual outcomes. In contrast to the outpatient setting, data suggests that in the inpatient setting, patients are able to accurately recall adverse events (Weingart et al. 2005; Weissman et al. 2008). Receipt of opioids was not related to satisfaction

(Mazurenko et al. 2019), but QoL was related to satisfaction in an older study (Larson et al. 1996). In a large multicenter study, missed nursing care was associated with lower satisfaction (Lake, Germack, and Viscardi 2016), and poor nurse-patient communication was associated with increased readmissions (Flanagan et al. 2016).

Heart disease is a well-studied outcome of the association between inpatient outcomes and satisfaction. One often cited study shows patient satisfaction was associated with decreased mortality and guideline adherence in acute myocardial infarction (Glickman et al. 2010). In addition, patient report of their subjective care quality after discharge were associated with functional status at 3, 6, and 12 months (Fremont et al. 2001), and satisfaction at 6 months was associated with lower presence of anginal symptoms (Plomondon et al. 2008). Also in myocardial infarction, patient centered-ness is associated with a moderately lower risk of death at 1 year (Meterko et al. 2010). In heart failure patients, interestingly, patient satisfaction was associated with 30-day readmissions, but other quality measures were not (Dy et al. 2016). This is one of the few studies showing that patient satisfaction outperforms other quality measures in terms of patient outcomes. Poor nurse-patient communication is also associated with heart failure readmissions (Stamp et al. 2014).

In inpatient care, the body of data across many disease states seems to suggest patient experience is associated with quality, reduced readmissions, and possibly reduced mortality. One of the benefits of the research on inpatients and patient experience is that most studies use validated tools (either HCAHPS or Press-Ganey®). The data is mostly correlation, still, though, and prospective studies on improving satisfaction leading to other improved outcomes are lacking.

Emergency and Critical Care

Care in the Emergency Department (ED) is especially unique given lack of continuity, patient acuity, time constraints, and the social determinants of health. An interesting nuance of patient experience in the

ED is that only discharged patients get patient experience surveys about their emergency care, while patients admitted to the hospital are only given inpatient surveys. Given these issues, the American College of Emergency Physicians has put out a paper which recognized that "policymakers and hospital leadership have conflated satisfaction and quality where the association between a patient's perception of care and the technical quality of services rendered and subsequent effect on desired patient outcomes are not validated" and that "evidence validating an association between patient satisfaction and objective measures of quality of care is mixed and contradictory at best." They go on to advocate for validated patient experience metrics to be used as standalone measure and not conflated with other measures of quality (Farley et al. 2014).

Dissatisfaction with discharge instructions from the ED is associated with not filling prescriptions (Thomas et al. 1996), though the association is not universal as more than half of patients who were satisfied with their instructions did not adhere to important recommendations in one study (Gignon et al. 2014). One specific example in EDs showed high satisfaction but low medication adherence in patients treated for pelvic inflammatory disease (Anders et al. 2018). Several other studies have shown satisfaction was tied to pain relief while in the ED (Bhakta and Marco 2014; Downey and Zun 2010; Schwartz et al. 2014). While there is no objective data to suggest over-testing or over-treatment related to satisfaction in the ED, an informal survey of 717 emergency physicians by Emergency Physicians Monthly showed that 59% of respondents reported increased testing and 48% of health care providers reported altering medical treatment due to the potential for a negative report on a patient satisfaction survey (2010).

While satisfaction is not reliably associated with patient outcomes in the ED, wait times, crowding, and boarding (other aspects of patient experience) are well known to be associated with mortality (Byrne et al. 2018; Hoot and Aronsky 2008; Plunkett et al. 2011; Richardson 2006; Sprivulis et al. 2006). However, while sometimes thought to be associated with decreased satisfaction, the use of hallway beds is not associated with poorer outcomes (Viccellio et al. 2009). As expected, ED crowding is also associated with delays in care, specifically for myocardial infarction (Schull et al. 2004), hip fractures (Hwang et al. 2006), pain (Mills et al. 2009; Pines et al. 2008; Pines et al. 2010), pneumonia (Pines et al. 2007), and stroke (Chen et al. 2006). Another study showed crowding was associated with increased mortality and delays in pneumonia care and pain control but not in reperfusion for ST elevation myocardial infarction (Bernstein et al. 2009). In other types of myocardial infarction, though, crowding and wait times were associated with increased adverse events (Pines et al. 2009) and decreased guideline compliance (Diercks et al. 2007). Wait times for patients with chest pain were not associated with actual costs or length of stay, but potentially missed revenue/opportunity costs (Bayley et al. 2005).

Critical care patients are another unique population. Unfortunately, it is very difficult to study patient experience in the intensive care unit, as most patients are unable to communicate easily while in critical care. Therefore, the role of patient satisfaction in this care setting has not been well-studied. When balancing patient experience versus other objective measures of quality, critical care would be a setting where objective quality measures (e.g., mortality, nosocomial infections) clearly outweigh those of patient experience.

SURGICAL SPECIALTIES

Patient satisfaction with outcomes in surgical care is an important outcome, especially in elective procedures. However, there is great controversy among surgeons regarding using patient experience as a measure for reimbursement (Tsai, Orav, Jha 2015). Some surgeons argue that much of the care they provide is in the operating room and not visible to the frequently sedated patient and that other influences of patient satisfaction are largely out of their control.

In analysis of hospital data from surgery, patient satisfaction, though highly variable, was associated with increased efficiency and decreased length of stay (Tsai, Orav, Jha 2015). Patients with increased satisfaction also had higher process quality measures (Sacks et al. 2015), lower readmission rates, and lower surgical mortality (Tsai, Orav, Jha 2015), confirmed in a second study (Lobo Prabhu et al. 2018). One study showed association with satisfaction and lower surgical complications (Iannuzzi et al. 2015), but another study showed an association with lower mortality but not postoperative complications, quality measures, length of stay, patient safety measures, or readmissions (Tevis, Kennedy, and Kent 2015). Two other studies showed no relationship between satisfaction and mortality, though (Elliott et al. 2013; Sheetz et al. 2014). Also, in complex cancer surgery cases, satisfaction is associated with decreased mortality and improved objective quality (Mehta et al. 2020). Other studies have shown no relationship between patient experience and adherence to guidelines (Lyu et al. 2013) or surgical complications, though (Schmocker). Berkowitz et al. found patients satisfaction to be linearly associated with both postoperative complications and pain (2019). In cholecystectomy patients, satisfaction was associated with health status and decrease symptoms (Kane, Maciejewski, and Finch; Mclean et al. 2017).

Cardiothoracic and Vascular Surgery

Similar to general surgery, patient satisfaction in thoracic surgery is associated with postoperative complications and pain (Cairns et al. 2020). In lung cancer surgery, satisfaction was associated with shorter length of stay (Singer et al. 2019). In a unique study, online physician ratings in cardiac surgery were weakly associated with decreased mortality (Liu et al, 2016). In vascular surgery, satisfaction was associated with pain and not complications or length of stay (O'Brien, Ianuzzi, and Kahn 2013).

Facial and Plastic/Reconstructive Surgery

Plastic surgery, often elective, is highly influenced by patient experience given the esthetic nature of the majority of cases. In breast surgery, esthetic results are more closely related to patient satisfaction than postoperative complications (Waljee, Newman, and Alderman 2008). But, in a study in a plastic surgery residency, complications and satisfaction were linked (Koulaxouzidis et al. 2014). In nasal symptom surgery, satisfaction was associated with decreased postoperative symptoms and lower out of pocket costs for the surgery (Nassiri et al. 2020); whereas, cost was not associated with satisfaction in patients with tinnitus (Goldstein et al. 2015).

Anesthesiology

The American Society of Anesthesiologists put out a white paper on patient satisfaction that stated "Measurement of patient satisfaction remains one of the most challenging and sometime confusing tasks for anesthesiologists. While there are legitimate concerns about survey reliability and validity, it is increasingly clear that there is increasing demand from hospitals, patients and payers that anesthesiologists assess patient satisfaction with their clinical care and their service" (Mesrobian et al. 2020). A large study found no association with postoperative nausea and vomiting and anesthesiologist satisfaction (Pozdnyakova et al. 2019). In two Saudi Arabian studies, postoperative symptoms (pain and nausea/vomiting) were related to satisfaction (Alsaif et al. 2018; Alshehri et al. 2015), and in an Australian study, satisfaction was associated with intraoperative awareness, postoperative pain, and postoperative nausea and vomiting (Myles et al. 2000). Satisfaction did not seem to be associated quality of recovery in another study, though (Berning et al. 2017).

Trauma and Orthopedics

Trauma patients are considered "high risk" for low satisfaction by some hospital leaders, but this is not supported by evidence (Bentley-Kumar et al. 2016). In trauma surgery, satisfaction is not associated with readmissions or mortality (Joseph et al. 2017; Thoma-Perry et al. 2018), but it is related to lower rates of postoperative complications in one study (Rogers et al. 2013) but not another (Joseph et al. 2017). In a small study, satisfaction was associated with shorter lengths of stay (Widger et al. 2003), as was a collaborative communication style of physicians (Chen et al. 2018).

In orthopedics, in particular, inadequate pain control is associated with decreased satisfaction, but increasing use of opioids is also associated with low satisfaction (Nota et al. 2015), specifically after fracture repair (Bot et al. 2014; Helmerhorst et al. 2012). Though, one study showed no difference between opioids and satisfaction in ankle fractures. (Finger et al. 2017) Orthopedic patients with a hospital acquired condition did not have different satisfaction scores than those who did not (Day et al. 2014).

Joint surgery is one of the most common elective surgeries in orthopedics. In patients undergoing knee or hip replacement, postoperative pain (in addition to preoperative expectations) was the factor most associated with satisfaction (Anakwe, Jenkins, and Moran 2011; Brokelman et al. 2020; Chugtai et al. 2016; Hamilton et al. 2013; Mistry et al. 2016; Mohamed et al. 2020), and in shoulder surgery, improvement in function (again, in addition to preoperative expectations) was most associated with satisfaction (Tashjian et al. 2007). One study did show no correlation between functional status and satisfaction in patients having hip replacement (Chugtai et al. 2018). Mancuso et al. (1997) showed that satisfaction was a complex phenomenon but was influenced by postoperative functional status (and preoperative expectations). In another study on patients undergoing hip replacement, though, postoperative pain and complications were not associated with complications (Patel et al.2017). Interestingly, while postoperative pain is associated with satisfaction, two studies showed receipt of opioid pain medications in the immediate postoperative period is associated with decreased satisfaction (Husted et al. 2008; Maher et al. 2016) but two others did not (Etcheson et al. 2018a; Etcheson et al. 2018b). Length of stay was not associated with satisfaction in one large study (Delanois et al. 2017), but in patients undergoing "fast track" surgery, length of stay was associated with several aspects of satisfaction including satisfaction with overall stay (Husted et al. 2008). A study on Press-Ganey® scores showed no association with knee-replacement specific outcomes reported by patients (Chughtai et al. 2017), and patient reported outcomes in joint replacement in general was also not associated with Press-Ganey® scores (Kohring et al. 2018). Inpatient satisfaction was not associated with cost or functional status in a large Medicaid database (Fisher et al. 2003). It also was not associated with postoperative complications at one institution (Mistry et al. 2017).

Spine and Neurosurgery

In general neurosurgery, satisfaction scores were also almost perfectly negatively correlated with quality, meaning lower quality was associated with higher satisfaction (Olivero et al. 2018). In cranial neurosurgery, satisfaction was associated with functional status and postoperative symptoms but not complications other than lower rates of minor infection (Reponen et al. 2015).

In patients undergoing several different types of spine surgery, postoperative pain control, postoperative complications, and postoperative function was associated with satisfaction in many studies (Hopkins et al. 2019a; Levin et al. 2017; Menendez et al. 2019; Mets et al. 2020). There was also a weak relationship between satisfaction and patient reported clinical outcome at 3 months (Bourne et al. 2017). It is also associated with shorter length of stay (Hopkins et al. 2019b; Smith et al. 2019; Mets et al. 2020), and highly associated with post-discharge emergency department visits (Smith et al. 2019) and readmission (Mets et al. 2020). However, in fusion surgery, kyphosis, and scoliosis, radiologic improvement was not associated with satisfaction (Berven et al. 2001; Kaptain et al. 2000;

Schiffman et al. 2003), but in scoliosis, postoperative flexibility was associated with satisfaction (Newton et al. 2009). In degenerative spine disease, functional outcome was associated with satisfaction (Mannion et al. 2009). In lumbar micro-diskectomy, length of stay was not associated with satisfaction (Lorish et al. 1998). In surgical treatment for cervical myelopathy, satisfaction was associated with improved health-related QoL (Doi et al. 2019).

Urology and Obstetrics and Gynecology

Obstetrics and gynecology and urology have extremely limited research on patient experience and health outcomes. Patients who rate quality of communication with their obstetrician high are more likely to maintain contraceptive use at 6 months (Dehlendorf et al. 2016). Patient perceptions of better communication and relationships with their midwives are associated with increased self-care behaviors during pregnancy (Nicoloro-SantaBarbara et al. 2017).

In urology, satisfaction is associated with patient reported treatment outcome (Schoenfelder et al. 2014). In urologic cancer surgery, there was no association between satisfaction and objective patient outcomes (Shirk et al. 2016), but a larger study in gynecologic cancer surgery showed higher satisfaction was associated with lower mortality and lower rates of surgical complications (Dottino et al. 2019).

In summarizing the data on the association between surgical care outcomes and patient experience, it is highly dependent on type of surgery and, even then, highly variable. In elective surgery, whether cosmetic or functional, the argument for patient satisfaction as a standalone measure is intuitively the strongest. Postoperative pain, postoperative complications, and prolonged length of stay seem to be most often associated with lower patient satisfaction across many surgery types. Interestingly, much data shows increased receipt of opioids postoperatively seems to correlate with lower satisfaction. In anesthesia care, patient satisfaction is mildly associated with uncontrolled symptoms like pain and nausea/vomiting. A couple of large studies on general surgical patients showed decreased mortality, though this outcome was not universally associated. It appears as though there is moderate, though inconsistent, correlation with patient satisfaction and some surgical outcomes. However, it is important to recognize that the vast majority of these studies were retrospective or had subjective symptoms and satisfaction measured contemporaneously.

MEDICAL SPECIALTIES

Patient experience is also an important measure in several medical specialties. However, the evidence for correlation to improved outcomes is weak or nonexistent in most specialties. This is due to the fact that many validated tools are not tailored to the nuances of specialty care. Also, fewer patients and physicians in each specialty makes large sample sizes required for quality research difficult to obtain.

Cancer

Cancer care has become increasingly complex. Primary malignancy, treatment options, side effects, prognosis, and health status especially confound patient experience measures in cancer care. One study showed the intuitive relationship between cancer patients' perceived service quality and likelihood to recommend (Lis, Rodeghier, and Gupta 2011). Patient perceptions of quality are associated with survival in several cancer types: breast cancer (Gupta, Rodheiger, and Lis 2013a), colon cancer (Gupta, Lis, and Rodheiger 2013), lung cancer (Gupta, Rodheiger, and Lis 2013b), and pancreatic cancer (Gupta et al. 2012). The only factor associated with survival and patient satisfaction in lung cancer patients was perception of teams communicating with each other (Lis, Patel, and Gupta 2015). Despite these multiple positive associations, the same research group found that in prostate cancer, self-related health status was a stronger predictor of survival than satisfaction (Gupta, Patel, and Lis 2015), again highlighting the complexities of the nuances of cancer care and patient experience measures (Alessy, Luchtenborg, and Davies 2019).

The relationship between QoL measures and patient experience in cancer, too, is complex. In Chinese lung and liver cancer patients, patient satisfaction is associated with increased QoL (Wong and Fielding 2008). Satisfied cancer survivors, too, report higher health status and decrease health care utilization (Rai et al. 2018). In contrast, in the US, Germany, and Spain, associations between satisfaction and QoL were uniformly poor (Arrara et al. 2013; Kleeberg et al. 2005). In several studies of cancer patients, satisfaction was shown to be associated with baseline health status (Lis, Patel, and Gupta 2015; Suhonen et al. 2018) and baseline QoL (Lis et al. 2009), emphasizing the limitations of retrospective and observational studies in identifying outcomes associated with patient experience measures.

Neurology

In neurology care, several major disease processes have been studied. As with primary care, patients with chronic headache with higher satisfaction had higher medication adherence (Fitzpatrick and Hopkins 1981). On the contrary, patients with headache who were prescribed medication were more likely to be satisfied (Bekkelund and Salvesen 2002). Similarly, in patients seeking a second opinion with a neurologist, satisfaction was tied to higher rates of admission (Wijers et al. 2010). Satisfaction with inpatient stroke care is associated with mixed results: overall satisfaction is associated with increased costs, decreased readmissions and mortality, but satisfaction with discharge information is associated with increased mortality (Xiang, Xu, and Foraker 2017). Inpatient stroke satisfaction is also associated with improved functional outcome at 3 months (Asplund et al. 2009). Interestingly, Pound et al. (1999) demonstrated that satisfaction with stroke care was actually associated with amount of outpatient therapy and outpatient social services received.

Cardiology

Heart disease is a leading cause of mortality in the US. A large study of patient after a myocardial infarction showed inpatient satisfaction was associated with increase guideline adherence and decreased mortality (Glickman et al. 2010). Further, hospitals with low satisfaction also have low objective quality in acute coronary syndrome (Girotra, Cram, and Popescu 2012). Patient-provider communication in cardiovascular disease is also associated patient reported and objective quality, but increased costs and healthcare utilization (Okunrintemi et al. 2017). Patient satisfaction is also associated with lower 30-day readmissions in heart failure (Hussein and Qayyum 2015). Details regarding satisfaction and myocardial infraction outcomes are discussed earlier in this chapter.

Dermatology

Skin conditions (other than cancer) are rarely associated with mortality but can cause great suffering for patients. High satisfaction in psoriasis is associated with decreased symptom burden (Korman et al. 2015). In actinic keratosis, good patient-physician communication is associated with improved patient reported symptoms and adherence to treatment (Neri et al. 2019).

Gastroenterology

In gastroenterology, patient satisfaction did not correlate with other measures of quality in patients undergoing colonoscopy (Yadlapati, Gawron, and Keswani 2014). In celiac disease, patient satisfaction is associated with increased testing, but not QoL or symptom severity (Faye et al. 2018), and in inflammatory bowel disease, satisfaction is associated with adherence (Bager et al. 2016). In patients with dyspepsia and peptic ulcer disease, satisfaction is closely related to pain (Rabeneck et al. 2000), and an intervention to improve patient's involvement with their care was tied to improved symptoms at six to eight weeks (Greenfield, Kaplan, and Ware 1985). Further, good patient-physician communication in patients with liver disease is associated with increased cancer screening (Li et al. 2017).

Psychiatry

Psychiatry is perhaps one of the difficult specialties to measure patient satisfaction, largely due to patient-related factors and the interplay with underlying diagnoses and perceptions of quality and satisfaction (Desai, Stefanovics, and Roshenheck 2005; Hoff et al. 1999; Kavalniene et al. 2018; Wyshak and Barsky 1995). Interestingly, in inpatient psychiatry patients, satisfaction is associated with QoL and medication adherence (Zendjidjian et al. 2014). In patients with depression, satisfaction is associated with less medications prescribed (Kohler et al. 2015), but in general psychiatric inpatients, satisfaction is associated with the receipt of medications (Kelstrup et al. 1993). There is also decreased satisfaction among patients who experience side effects of medications prescribed (Gebhardt, Wolak, and Huber 2013). In outpatient care, receipt of quality psychiatric behavioral interventions (but not medication) is associated with increased satisfaction in patients with anxiety (Stein et al. 2011) and a better therapeutic alliance is associated with better functional outcomes with less medication in schizophrenia (Frank and Gunderson 1990).

Rheumatology

Rheumatology is an interesting specialty that deals with patients with chronic pain and symptoms often unexplained by other physicians. Agarwal et al. (2012) showed that satisfaction with rheumatology care predicted patient intention to return to care. This is not surprising given the contemporaneous measurement and subjective nature of both measures.

Satisfaction in fibromyalgia patients is associated with higher health care costs (Serber, Cronan, and Walen 2003), but patients who perceived poor treatment control visited the hospital fewer times, while patients who reported being discounted by medical professionals visited the hospital more times (Homma, Ishikawa, Kiuchi and 2018). Another study in patients with lupus and rheumatoid arthritis showed that trust in one's physician was associated with increased global health status and decreased medication side effects (Berios-Rivera et al. 2006). In a study on lupus alone, though, satisfaction with care was associated with increased symptoms burden (Jolly et al. 2019), but it was not associated with increased cost in another study (Sutcliffe et al. 2001). Satisfaction is associated with improved health related QoL in lupus (Dua et al. 2012). And, participatory communication between patients and physicians is associated with less organ damage (Ward et al. 2003).

CONCLUSION

This chapter summarizes the literature on patient experience and satisfaction measures and health outcomes. There is strong evidence for outpatient satisfaction and medication adherence and moderate evidence for diabetes care, though both using only surrogate measures. One large study showed increased mortality with increased outpatient satisfaction, and several others have shown potential for over-testing and over-treatment. The data for inpatient care points towards correlation between satisfaction and higher quality, decreased readmissions, and decreased mortality. In emergency medicine, there are no convincing associations with satisfaction and outcomes, but there is a strong association with wait times, crowding, and boarding and mortality and delays in care. In surgical care across most specialties, postoperative symptoms and complications are those most often correlated with low satisfaction. Two large studies showed decreased mortality with increased patient satisfaction, but two other studies did not. In medical specialties, there is limited data on associations with health outcomes and the data is largely specialty-specific.

It is important to understand the limitations of these studies. First, measurement of patient experience or satisfaction in these studies was quite heterogenous. Many studies only measure certain components of patient experience (i.e., satisfaction, communication). Only about half of the included studies were done using validated tools, and even less used the HCAHPS and other tools endorsed by CMS. The first step in science is collecting valid and reliable data. If experience is going to be tied to reimbursement, it is important that we use the tools that have the most robust evidence to support them.

Further, while there are many studies that show associations with health outcomes, nearly all of these studies were retrospective and correlational in nature. Several studies actually highlighted that relationships between satisfaction and outcome variables maybe the results of reverse causation. That is, the health outcome may have caused the poor satisfaction. This is especially relevant since many, though not all, studies measured outcomes either before or contemporaneously with satisfaction. For example, postoperative pain is measured in the hospital and satisfaction is measured after discharge and the former could affect the latter. There were no studies that showed interventions to improve satisfaction actually led to improved outcomes.

Patient experience, of course, may be considered a standalone quality measure. But, given its inconsistent associations with other outcomes, it is important to not use it in isolation. Patient experience should not be overemphasized without considering other balance measures to prevent affecting overall quality.

REFERENCES

Agency for Healthcare Research and Quality. 2017. *What Is Patient Experience?* Last modified March 2017. https://www.ahrq.gov/cahps/about-cahps/patient-experience/index.html.

Agnihotri, Kasturi, and Shally Awasthi. 2011. "Parental Reporting Of Quality Of Care As A Determinant Of Health Related Quality Of Life

Of Ill Adolescents At A Tertiary Care Hospital In Northern India." *The Indian Journal of Pediatrics* 79 (1): 62-67. doi:10.1007/s12098-011-0528-4.

Agrawal, Harsh, M. Cameron Hay, Elizabeth R. Volkmann, Paul Maranian, Dinesh Khanna, and Daniel E. Furst. 2012. "Satisfaction And Access To Clinical Care In A Rheumatology Clinic At A Large Urban Medical Center." *JCR: Journal of Clinical Rheumatology* 18 (4): 209-211. doi:10.1097/rhu.0b013e318259aa1b.

Alamo, Miguel Muñoz, Roger Ruiz Moral, and Luis Angel Pérula de Torres. 2002. "Evaluation Of A Patient-Centred Approach In Generalized Musculoskeletal Chronic Pain/Fibromyalgia Patients In Primary Care." *Patient Education and Counseling* 48 (1): 23-31. doi:10.1016/s0738-3991(02)00095-2.

Alessy, Saleh A., Margreet Lüchtenborg, and Elizabeth A. Davies. 2019. "How Have Patients' Experiences Of Cancer Care Been Linked To Survival? A Systematic Review." *Patient Experience Journal* 6 (1): 63-80. doi:10.35680/2372-0247.1323.

Alsaif, Abdulrahman, Saleh Alqahtani, Farhan Alanazi, Faris Alrashed, and Abdullah Almutairi. 2018. "Patient Satisfaction And Experience With Anesthesia: A Multicenter Survey In Saudi Population." *Saudi Journal of Anaesthesia* 12 (2): 304. doi:10.4103/sja.sja_656_17.

Al Shahrani, Abeer, and Muneera Baraja. 2014. "Patient Satisfaction And It'S Relation To Diabetic Control In A Primary Care Setting." *Journal of Family Medicine and Primary Care* 3 (1): 5. doi:10.4103/2249-4863.130254.

Alshehri, AdelAli, YasserMohammed Alomar, Ghali Abdulrahman Mohammed, Mazen Saud Al-Fozan, Mohammed Saleh Al-Harbi, Khalid Abduraziz Alrobai, and Haroon Zahoor. 2015. "A Survey On Postanesthetic Patient Satisfaction In A University Hospital." *Saudi Journal of Anaesthesia* 9 (3): 303. doi:10.4103/1658-354x.158499.

American Hospital Association. 2020. "Fast Facts on U.S. Hospitals, 2020." In *2020 AHA Hospital Statistics*. Chicago: The Association.

Amin, Suvina, Mena Soliman, Andrew McIvor, Andrew Cave, and Claudia Cabrera. 2020. "Understanding Patient Perspectives On Medication

Adherence In Asthma: A Targeted Review Of Qualitative Studies</P>." *Patient Preference and Adherence* Volume 14: 541-551. doi:10.2147/ppa.s234651.

Anakwe, Raymond E., Paul J. Jenkins, and Matthew Moran. 2011. "Predicting Dissatisfaction After Total Hip Arthroplasty: A Study Of 850 Patients." *The Journal of Arthroplasty* 26 (2): 209-213. doi:10.1016/j.arth.2010.03.013.

Anbori, A., S. N. Ghani, H. Yadav, A. M. Daher, and T. T. Su. 2010. "Patient Satisfaction And Loyalty To The Private Hospitals In Sana'a, Yemen." *International Journal for Quality in Health Care* 22 (4): 310-315. doi:10.1093/intqhc/mzq029.

Anders, Jennifer, Alexandra Hill, Shang-En Chung, Arlene Butz, Richard Rothman, Charlotte Gaydos, Jamie Perin, and Maria Trent. 2017. "Patient Satisfaction And Treatment Adherence For Urban Adolescents And Young Adults With Pelvic Inflammatory Disease." *Trauma and Emergency Care* 3 (1). doi:10.15761/tec.1000152.

Arbuthnott, Alexis, and Donald Sharpe. 2009. "The Effect Of Physician–Patient Collaboration On Patient Adherence In Non-Psychiatric Medicine." *Patient Education and Counseling* 77 (1): 60-67. doi:10.1016/j.pec.2009.03.022.

Arraras, Juan Ignacio, Jose Juan Illarramendi, Antonio Viudez, Berta Ibáñez, Maria Jose Lecumberri, Susana de la Cruz, and Berta Hernandez et al. 2013. "Determinants Of Patient Satisfaction With Care In A Spanish Oncology Day Hospital And Its Relationship With Quality Of Life." *Psycho-Oncology* 22 (11): 2454-2461. doi:10.1002/pon.3307.

Asadi-Lari, Mohsen, Chris Packham, and David Gray. 2003. *Health and Quality of Life Outcomes* 1 (1): 57. doi:10.1186/1477-7525-1-57.

Asplund, Kjell, Fredrik Jonsson, Marie Eriksson, Birgitta Stegmayr, Peter Appelros, Bo Norrving, Andreas Terént, and Kerstin Hulter Åsberg. 2009. "Patient Dissatisfaction With Acute Stroke Care." *Stroke* 40 (12): 3851-3856. doi:10.1161/strokeaha.109.561985.

Australian Commission on Safety and Quality in HealthCare. 2012. *Review of patient experience and satisfaction surveys conducted within public* and private hospitals in Australia. Last modified May 5, 2012. https://www.safetyandquality.gov.au/sites/default/files/migrated/Review-of-Hospital-Patient-Experience-Surveys-conducted-by-Australian-Hospitals-30-March-2012-FINAL.pdf.

Bager, Palle, Mette Julsgaard, Thea Vestergaard, Lisbet Ambrosius Christensen, and Jens Frederik Dahlerup. 2016. "Adherence And Quality Of Care In IBD." *Scandinavian Journal of Gastroenterology* 51 (11): 1326-1331. doi:10.1080/00365521.2016.1195870.

Bakar, Zanariah Abu, Mathumalar Loganathan Fahrni, and Tahir Mehmood Khan. 2016. "Patient Satisfaction And Medication Adherence Assessment Amongst Patients At The Diabetes Medication Therapy Adherence Clinic." *Diabetes & Metabolic Syndrome: Clinical Research & Reviews* 10 (2): S139-S143. doi:10.1016/j.dsx.2016.03.015.

Bardach, Naomi S, Renée Asteria-Peñaloza, W John Boscardin, and R Adams Dudley. 2012. "The Relationship Between Commercial Website Ratings And Traditional Hospital Performance Measures In The USA." *BMJ Quality & Safety* 22 (3): 194-202. doi:10.1136/bmjqs-2012-001360.

Barnes, Camilla B., and Charlotte S. Ulrik. 2014. "Asthma And Adherence To Inhaled Corticosteroids: Current Status And Future Perspectives." *Respiratory Care* 60 (3): 455-468. doi:10.4187/respcare.03200.

Bayley, Matthew D., J. Sanford Schwartz, Frances S. Shofer, Mark Weiner, Frank D. Sites, K. Bobbi Traber, and Judd E. Hollander. 2005. "The Financial Burden Of Emergency Department Congestion And Hospital Crowding For Chest Pain Patients Awaiting Admission." *Annals of Emergency Medicine* 45 (2): 110-117. doi:10.1016/j.annemergmed.2004.09.010.

Beattie, Michelle, Douglas J. Murphy, Iain Atherton, and William Lauder. 2015. "Instruments To Measure Patient Experience Of Healthcare Quality In Hospitals: A Systematic Review." *Systematic Reviews* 4 (1). doi:10.1186/s13643-015-0089-0.

Bekkelund, Svein Ivar, and Rolf Salvesen. 2002. "Patient Satisfaction With A Neurological Specialist Consultation For Headache." *Scandinavian*

Journal of Primary Health Care 20 (3): 157-160. doi:10.1080/028134302760234609.

Bentley-Kumar, Karalyn, Theresa Jackson, Danny Holland, Brian LeBlanc, Vaidehi Agrawal, and Michael S. Truitt. 2016. "Trauma Patients: I Can't Get No (Patient) Satisfaction?" *The American Journal of Surgery* 212 (6): 1256-1260. doi:10.1016/j.amjsurg.2016.09.023.

Berkowitz, Rachel, Joceline Vu, Chad Brummett, Jennifer Waljee, Michael Englesbe, and Ryan Howard. 2019. "The Impact Of Complications And Pain On Patient Satisfaction." *Annals of Surgery* Publish Ahead of Print. doi:10.1097/sla.0000000000003621.

Berning, V., Martin Laupheimer, Matthias Nübling, and Thomas Heidegger. 2017. "Influence Of Quality Of Recovery On Patient Satisfaction With Anaesthesia And Surgery: A Prospective Observational Cohort Study." *Anaesthesia* 72 (9): 1088-1096. doi:10.1111/anae.13906.

Bernstein, Steven L., Dominik Aronsky, Reena Duseja, Stephen Epstein, Dan Handel, Ula Hwang, and Melissa McCarthy et al. 2009. "The Effect Of Emergency Department Crowding On Clinically Oriented Outcomes." *Academic Emergency Medicine* 16 (1): 1-10. doi:10.1111/j.1553-2712.2008.00295.x.

Berrios-Rivera, Javier P., Richard L. Street, Maria G. Garcia Popa-lisseanu, Michael A. Kallen, Marsha N. Richardson, Namieta M. Janssen, Donald M. Marcus, John D. Reveille, Noranna B. Warner, and Maria E. Suarez-almazor. 2006. "Trust In Physicians And Elements Of The Medical Interaction In Patients With Rheumatoid Arthritis And Systemic Lupus Erythematosus." *Arthritis & Rheumatism* 55 (3): 385-393. doi:10.1002/art.21988.

Berven, Sigurd H., Vedat Deviren, Jason A. Smith, Arash Emami, Serena S. Hu, and David S. Bradford. 2001. "Management Of Fixed Sagittal Plane Deformity." *Spine* 26 (18): 2036-2043. doi:10.1097/00007632-200109150-00020.

Berwick, Donald M. 2009. "What 'Patient-Centered' Should Mean: Confessions Of An Extremist." *Health Affairs* 28 (Supplement 1): w555-w565. doi:10.1377/hlthaff.28.4.w555.

Bhakta, Hemangini C., and Catherine A. Marco. 2014. "Pain Management: Association With Patient Satisfaction Among Emergency Department Patients." *The Journal of Emergency Medicine* 46 (4): 456-464. doi:10.1016/j.jemermed.2013.04.018.

Billinghurst, Brenda, Michael Whitfield. 1993. "Why do patients change their general practitioner? A postal questionnaire study of patients in Avon." *British Journal of General Practice*. 43 (373): 336-338.

Bjertnaes, Oyvind, Hilde Hestad Iversen, Katrine Damgaard Skyrud, and Kirsten Danielsen. 2019. "The Value Of Facebook In Nation-Wide Hospital Quality Assessment: A National Mixed-Methods Study In Norway." *BMJ Quality & Safety* 29 (3): 217-224. doi:10.1136/bmjqs-2019-009456.

Bot, Arjan G. J., Stijn Bekkers, Paul M. Arnstein, R. Malcolm Smith, and David Ring. 2014. "Opioid Use After Fracture Surgery Correlates With Pain Intensity And Satisfaction With Pain Relief." *Clinical Orthopaedics and Related Research®* 472 (8): 2542-2549. doi:10.1007/s11999-014-3660-4.

Bottle, Alex, Christopher Tsang, Camille Parsons, Azeem Majeed, Michael Soljak, and Paul Aylin. 2012. "Association Between Patient And General Practice Characteristics And Unplanned First-Time Admissions For Cancer: Observational Study." *British Journal of Cancer* 107 (8): 1213-1219. doi:10.1038/bjc.2012.320.

Boulding, William, Seth W. Glickman, Matthew P. Manary, Kevin A. Schulman, and Richard Staelin, R. 2011. "Relationship between patient satisfaction with inpatient care and hospital readmission within 30 days." *The American Journal of Managed Care 17* (1): 41–48.

Bourne, James T., Charlotte E. Cross, Irfan N. Yasin, and Mohammed N. Yasin. 2017. "Surgical Outcomes And Healthcare Experience In Spinal Surgery: Are They Related." *Orthopedics and Rheumatology Open Access Journal* 7 (1). doi:10.19080/oroaj.2017.07.555701.

Brokelman, Roy B. G., Daniel Haverkamp, Corné van Loon, Annemiek Hol, Albert van Kampen, and Rene Veth. 2012. "The Validation Of The Visual Analogue Scale For Patient Satisfaction After Total Hip

Arthroplasty." *European Orthopaedics and Traumatology* 3 (2): 101-105. doi:10.1007/s12570-012-0100-3.

Byrne, Declan, Joseph Browne, Richard Conway, Sean Cournane, Deidre O'Riordanand Bernard Silke, Bernard. 2018. "Mortality outcomes and emergency department wait times - the paradox in the capacity limited system." *Acute medicine* 17 (3): 130-136.

Cabana, Michael D., Kathryn K. Slish, David Evans, Robert B. Mellins, Randall W. Brown, Xihong Lin, Niko Kaciroti, and Noreen M. Clark. 2014. "Impact Of Physician Asthma Care Education On Patient Outcomes." *Health Education & Behavior* 41 (5): 509-517. doi:10.1177/1090198114547510.

Calderon-Larranaga, Amaia, Leanne Carney, Michael Soljak, Alex Bottle, Martyn Partridge, Derek Bell, Gerrard Abi-Aad, Paul Aylin, and Azeem Majeed. 2010. "Association Of Population And Primary Healthcare Factors With Hospital Admission Rates For Chronic Obstructive Pulmonary Disease In England: National Cross-Sectional Study." *Thorax* 66 (3): 191-196. doi:10.1136/thx.2010.147058.

Calderón-Larrañaga, Amaia, Michael Soljak, Elizabeth Cecil, Jonathan Valabhji, Derek Bell, A.lexandra Prados Torres, and Azeem Majeed. 2014. "Does Higher Quality Of Primary Healthcare Reduce Hospital Admissions For Diabetes Complications? A National Observational Study." *Diabetic Medicine* 31 (6): 657-665. doi:10.1111/dme.12413.

Calderón-Larrañaga, Amaia, Michael Soljak, Thomas E. Cowling, Athanasios Gaitatzis, and Azeem Majeed. 2014. "Association Of Primary Care Factors With Hospital Admissions For Epilepsy In England, 2004–2010: National Observational Study." *Seizure* 23 (8): 657-661. doi:10.1016/j.seizure.2014.05.008.

Cairns, Alexander, Finn McLennan Battleday, Galina Velikova, Alessandro Brunelli, Heather Bell, Joel Favo, Miriam Patella, Oana Lindner, and Cecilia Pompili. 2020. "General Patient Satisfaction After Elective And Acute Thoracic Surgery Is Associated With Postoperative Complications." *Journal of Thoracic Disease* 12 (5): 2088-2095. doi:10.21037/jtd-19-3345b.

Campbell, Lauren, and Yue Li. 2017. "Are Facebook User Ratings Associated With Hospital Cost, Quality And Patient Satisfaction? A Cross-Sectional Analysis Of Hospitals In New York State." *BMJ Quality & Safety* 27 (2): 119-129. doi:10.1136/bmjqs-2016-006291.

Carcaise-Edinboro, Patricia, and Cathy J. Bradley. 2008. "Influence of Patient-Provider Communication on Colorectal Cancer Screening." *Medical Care* 46 (7): 738–745. https://doi.org/10.1097/mlr.0b013e318178935a.

Carrico, Jacqueline A., Katharine Mahoney, Kristen M. Raymond, Logan Mims, Peter C. Smith, Joseph T. Sakai, Susan K. Mikulich-Gilbertson, Christian J. Hopfer, and Karsten Bartels. 2018. "The Association Of Patient Satisfaction-Based Incentives With Primary Care Physician Opioid Prescribing." *The Journal of The American Board of Family Medicine* 31 (6): 941-943. doi:10.3122/jabfm.2018.06.180067.

Cecil, Elizabeth, Alex Bottle, T.homas E. Cowling, Azeem Majeed, Ingrid Wolfe, and Sonia Saxena. 2016. "Primary Care Access, Emergency Department Visits, And Unplanned Short Hospitalizations In The UK." *Pediatrics* 137 (2): e20151492-e20151492. doi:10.1542/peds.2015-1492.

Centers for Disease Control and Prevention. 2017. "Faststats." Last modified January 19, 2017. https://www.cdc.gov/nchs/fastats/physician-visits.htm.

Center for Medicare and Medicaid Services. 2020. *HCAHPS: Patients' Perspectives Of Care Survey | CMS*. Last modified February 11, 2020. http://www.cms.gov/Medicare/Quality-Initiatives-Patient-Assessment-Instruments/HospitalQualityInits/HospitalHCAHPS.html.

Cerier, Emily, Eliza W. Beal, Jeffery Chakedis, Qinyu Chen, Anghela Paredes, Steven Sun, Jordan M. Cloyd, and Timothy M. Pawlik. 2018. "Patient-Provider Relationships And Health Outcomes Among Hepatopancreatobiliary Patients." *Journal of Surgical Research* 228: 290-298. doi:10.1016/j.jss.2018.03.026.

Chang, John T., Ron D. Hays, Paul G. Shekelle, Catherine H. MacLean, David H. Solomon, David B. Reuben, and Carol P. Roth et al. 2006. "Patients' Global Ratings Of Their Health Care Are Not Associated

With The Technical Quality Of Their Care." *Annals of Internal Medicine* 144 (9): 665. doi:10.7326/0003-4819-144-9-200605020-00010.

Cheiloudaki, Emmanouela, and Evangelos Alexopoulos. 2019. "Adherence To Treatment In Stroke Patients." *International Journal of Environmental Research and Public Health* 16 (2): 196. doi:10.3390/ijerph16020196.

Chen, Alissa, Frances Lee Revere, and Chris Beck. 2017. "Evaluation Of Quality Outcomes And HCAHPS Scores Between Academic And Non-Academic Hospitals." *Academy of Management Proceedings* 2017 (1): 15977. doi:10.5465/ambpp.2017.15977abstract.

Chen, Esther H., Angela M. Mills, Bruce Y. Lee, Jennifer L. Robey, Kara E. Zogby, Frances S. Shofer, Patrick M. Reilly, and Judd E. Hollander. 2006. "The Impact Of A Concurrent Trauma Alert Evaluation On Time To Head Computed Tomography In Patients With Suspected Stroke." *Academic Emergency Medicine* 13 (3): 349-352. doi:10.1197/j.aem.2005.10.011.

Chen, Pei-Ching, Yue-Chune Lee, and Raymond Nienchen Kuo. 2012. "Differences In Patient Reports On The Quality Of Care In A Diabetes Pay-For-Performance Program Between 1 Year Enrolled And Newly Enrolled Patients." *International Journal for Quality in Health Care* 24 (2): 189-196. doi:10.1093/intqhc/mzr091.

Chen, Qinyu, Eliza W. Beal, Eric B. Schneider, Victor Okunrintemi, Xufeng Zhang, and Timothy M. Pawlik. 2017. "Patient-Provider Communication And Health Outcomes Among Individuals With Hepato-Pancreato-Biliary Disease In The USA." *Journal of Gastrointestinal Surgery* 22 (4): 624-632. doi:10.1007/s11605-017-3610-z.

Chen, Qinyu, Eliza W. Beal, Victor Okunrintemi, Emily Cerier, Anghela Paredes, Steven Sun, Griffin Olsen, and Timothy M. Pawlik. 2018. "The Association Between Patient Satisfaction And Patient-Reported Health Outcomes." *Journal of Patient Experience* 6 (3): 201-209. doi:10.1177/2374373518795414.

Chen, You, Mayur B. Patel, Candace D. McNaughton, and Bradley A. Malin. 2018. "Interaction Patterns Of Trauma Providers Are Associated With Length Of Stay." *Journal of The American Medical Informatics Association* 25 (7): 790-799. doi:10.1093/jamia/ocy009.

Chughtai, Morad, Chukwuweike U. Gwam, Anton Khlopas, Nipun Sodhi, Ronald E. Delanois, Kurt P. Spindler, and Michael A. Mont. 2018. "No Correlation Between Press Ganey Survey Responses And Outcomes In Post–Total Hip Arthroplasty Patients." *The Journal of Arthroplasty* 33 (3): 783-785. doi:10.1016/j.arth.2017.09.037.

Chughtai, Morad, Julio J. Jauregui, Jaydev B. Mistry, Randa K. Elmallah, Aloise M. Diedrich, Peter M. Bonutti, Ronald Delanois, and Michael A. 2016. "What Influences How Patients Rate Their Hospital After Total Knee Arthroplasty?" *Surgical Technology International* 28: 261–265.

Chughtai, Morad, Nirav K. Patel, Chukwuweike U. Gwam, Anton Khlopas, Peter M. Bonutti, Ronald E. Delanois, and Michael A. Mont. 2017. "Do Press Ganey Scores Correlate With Total Knee Arthroplasty—Specific Outcome Questionnaires In Postsurgical Patients?" *The Journal of Arthroplasty* 32 (9): S109-S112. doi:10.1016/j.arth.2017.01.007.

Cinar, Ayse Basak, and Lone Schou. 2014. "Interrelation Between Patient Satisfaction And Patient-Provider Communication In Diabetes Management." *The Scientific World Journal* 2014: 1-8. doi:10.1155/2014/372671.

Clark, Noreen M., Michael D. Cabana, Bin Nan, Z. Molly Gong, Kathryn K. Slish, Nancy A. Birk, and Niko Kaciroti. 2007. "The Clinician-Patient Partnership Paradigm: Outcomes Associated With Physician Communication Behavior." *Clinical Pediatrics* 47 (1): 49-57. doi:10.1177/0009922807305650.

Cowling, Thomas E., Azeem Majeed, and Matthew J. Harris. 2018. "Patient Experience Of General Practice And Use Of Emergency Hospital Services In England: Regression Analysis Of National Cross-Sectional Time Series Data." *BMJ Quality & Safety* 27 (8): 643-654. doi:10.1136/bmjqs-2017-007174.

Cowling, Thomas E., Elizabeth V. Cecil, Michael A. Soljak, John Tayu Lee, Christopher Millett, Azeem Majeed, Robert M. Wachter, and Matthew J. Harris. 2013. "Access To Primary Care And Visits To Emergency Departments In England: A Cross-Sectional, Population-Based Study." *Plos ONE* 8 (6): e66699. doi:10.1371/journal.pone.0066699.

D'Agostino, Ralph B. 2000. "Debate: The Slippery Slope Of Surrogate Outcomes." *Trials* 1 (2). doi:10.1186/cvm-1-2-076.

Day, Michael S., Lorraine H. Hutzler, Raj Karia, Kella Vangsness, Nina Setia, and Joseph A. Bosco. 2014. "Hospital-Acquired Conditions After Orthopedic Surgery Do Not Affect Patient Satisfaction Scores." *Journal for Healthcare Quality* 36 (6): 33-40. doi:10.1111/jhq.12031.

Dehlendorf, Christine, Jillian T. Henderson, Eric Vittinghoff, Kevin Grumbach, Kira Levy, Julie Schmittdiel, Jennifer Lee, Dean Schillinger, and Jody Steinauer. 2016. "Association Of The Quality Of Interpersonal Care During Family Planning Counseling With Contraceptive Use." *Obstetrical & Gynecological Survey* 71 (6): 342-343. doi:10.1097/01.ogx.0000483079.25754.3d.

Delanois, Ronald E., Chukwuweike U. Gwam, Jaydev B. Mistry, Morad Chughtai, Anton Khlopas, George Yakubek, Prem N. Ramkumar, Nicolas S. Piuzzi, and Michael A. Mont. 2018. "Does Gender Influence How Patients Rate Their Patient Experience After Total Hip Arthroplasty?" *HIP International* 28 (1): 40-43. doi:10.5301/hipint.5000510.

Desai, Rani A., Elina A. Stefanovics, and Robert A. Rosenheck. 2005. "The Role Of Psychiatric Diagnosis In Satisfaction With Primary Care." *Medical Care* 43 (12): 1208-1216. doi:10.1097/01.mlr.0000185747.79104.90.

Diercks, Deborah B., Matthew T. Roe, Anita Y. Chen, W. Franklin Peacock, J. Douglas Kirk, Charles V. Pollack, W. Brian Gibler, Sidney C. Smith, Magnus Ohman, and Eric D. Peterson. 2007. "Prolonged Emergency Department Stays Of Non–ST-Segment-Elevation Myocardial Infarction Patients Are Associated With Worse Adherence To The American College Of Cardiology/American Heart Association

Guidelines For Management And Increased Adverse Events." *Annals of Emergency Medicine* 50 (5): 489-496. doi:10.1016/j.annemergmed. 2007.03.033.

Doi, Toru, Hideki Nakamoto, Koji Nakajima, Shima Hirai, Yusuke Sato, So Kato, and Yuki Taniguchi et al. 2019. "Effect Of Depression And Anxiety On Health-Related Quality Of Life Outcomes And Patient Satisfaction After Surgery For Cervical Compressive Myelopathy." *Journal of Neurosurgery: Spine* 31 (6): 816-823. doi:10.3171/2019.6.spine19569.

Downey, La VonneA, and LeslieS Zun. 2010. "Pain Management In The Emergency Department And Its Relationship To Patient Satisfaction." *Journal of Emergencies, Trauma, And Shock* 3 (4): 326. doi:10.4103/0974-2700.70749.

Doyle, Cathal, Laura Lennox, and Derek Bell. 2013. "A Systematic Review Of Evidence On The Links Between Patient Experience And Clinical Safety And Effectiveness." *BMJ Open* 3 (1): e001570. doi:10.1136/bmjopen-2012-001570.

Dragovich, Anthony, Thomas Beltran, George M. Baylor, Marc Swanson, and Anthony Plunkett. 2017. "Determinants Of Patient Satisfaction In A Private Practice Pain Management Clinic." *Pain Practice* 17 (8): 1015-1022. doi:10.1111/papr.12554.

Dua, Anisha B., Rohit Aggarwal, Rachel A. Mikolaitis, Winston Sequeira, Joel A. Block, and Meenakshi Jolly. 2012. "Rheumatologist's Quality Of Care For Lupus: Comparison Study Between A University And County Hospital." *Arthritis Care & Research*, n/a-n/a. doi:10.1002/acr.21653.

Dy, Sydney Morss, Kitty S. Chan, Hsien-Yen Chang, Allen Zhang, Junya Zhu, and Deirdre Mylod. 2016. "Patient Perspectives Of Care And Process And Outcome Quality Measures For Heart Failure Admissions In US Hospitals: How Are They Related In The Era Of Public Reporting?" *International Journal for Quality in Health Care* 28 (4): 522-528. doi:10.1093/intqhc/mzw063.

Elliott, Marc N., Amelia M. Haviland, Paul D. Cleary, Alan M. Zaslavsky, Donna O. Farley, David J. Klein, Carol A. Edwards, Megan K.

Beckett, Nate Orr, and Debra Saliba. 2013. "Care Experiences Of Managed Care Medicare Enrollees Near The End Of Life." *Journal of The American Geriatrics Society* 61 (3): 407-412. doi:10.1111/jgs.12121.

Emergency Physicans Monthly. 2010. *2+2=7? Seven Things You May Not Know About Press Ganey Statistics*. Last modified 2019. https://epmonthly.com/article/227-seven-things-you-may-not-know-about-press-gainey-statistics/.

Emmert, Martin, Thomas Adelhardt, Uwe Sander, Veit Wambach, and Jörg Lindenthal. 2015. "A Cross-Sectional Study Assessing The Association Between Online Ratings And Structural And Quality Of Care Measures: Results From Two German Physician Rating Websites." *BMC Health Services Research* 15 (1). doi:10.1186/s12913-015-1051-5.

Etcheson, Jennifer I., Chukwuweike U. Gwam, Nicole E. George, Alexander T. Caughran, Michael A. Mont, and Ronald E. Delanois. 2018. "Does The Amount Of Opioid Consumed Influence How Patients Rate Their Experience Of Care After Total Knee Arthroplasty?" *The Journal of Arthroplasty* 33 (11): 3407-3411. doi:10.1016/j.arth.2018.06.028.

Etcheson, Jennifer I., Chukwuweike U. Gwam, Nicole E. George, Sana Virani, Michael A. Mont, and Ronald E. Delanois. 2018. "Opioids Consumed In The Immediate Post-Operative Period Do Not Influence How Patients Rate Their Experience Of Care After Total Hip Arthroplasty." *The Journal of Arthroplasty* 33 (4): 1008-1011. doi:10.1016/j.arth.2017.10.033.

Farley, Heather, Enrique R. Enguidanos, Christian M. Coletti, Leah Honigman, Anthony Mazzeo, Thomas B. Pinson, Kevin Reed, and Jennifer L. Wiler. 2014. "Patient Satisfaction Surveys And Quality Of Care: An Information Paper." *Annals of Emergency Medicine* 64 (4): 351-357. doi:10.1016/j.annemergmed.2014.02.021.

Faye, Adam, Srihari Mahadev, Benjamin Lebwohl, and Peter Green. 2016. "Determinants Of Patient Satisfaction With Medical Care In Celiac

Disease." *American Journal of Gastroenterology* 111: S459-S460. doi:10.14309/00000434-201610001-01058.

Fenton, Joshua J., Anthony F. Jerant, Klea D. Bertakis, Peter Franks. 2012. "The Cost Of Satisfaction." *Archives of Internal Medicine* 172 (5): 405. doi:10.1001/archinternmed.2011.1662.

Finger, Abigail, Teun Teunis, Michiel G. Hageman, Emily R. Ziady, David Ring, and Marilyn Heng. 2017. "Association Between Opioid Intake And Disability After Surgical Management Of Ankle Fractures." *Journal of The American Academy Of Orthopaedic Surgeons* 25 (7): 519-526. doi:10.5435/jaaos-d-16-00505.

Fisher, Elliott S., David E. Wennberg, Thrse A. Stukel, Daniel J. Gottlieb, F. L. Lucas, and Étoile L. Pinder. 2003. "The Implications Of Regional Variations In Medicare Spending. Part 2: Health Outcomes And Satisfaction With Care." *Annals of Internal Medicine* 138 (4): 288. doi:10.7326/0003-4819-138-4-200302180-00007.

Fitzpatrick, Ray M., and Anthony Hopkins. 1981. "Patients' Satisfaction With Communication In Neurological Outpatient Clinics." *Journal of Psychosomatic Research* 25 (5): 329-334. doi:10.1016/0022-3999(81)90043-x.

Flanagan, Jane, Kelly D. Stamp, Matt Gregas, and Judy Shindul-Rothschild. 2016. "Predictors Of 30-Day Readmission For Pneumonia." *JONA: The Journal of Nursing Administration* 46 (2): 69-74. doi:10.1097/nna.0000000000000297.

Fortuna, Robert J., Angela K. Nagel, Thomas A. Rocco, Sharon Legette-Sobers, and Denise D. Quigley. 2017. "Patient Experience With Care And Its Association With Adherence To Hypertension Medications." *American Journal of Hypertension* 31 (3): 340-345. doi:10.1093/ajh/hpx200.

Frank, Arlene F., and John G. Gunderson. 1990. "The Role Of The Therapeutic Alliance In The Treatment Of Schizophrenia." *Archives of General Psychiatry* 47 (3): 228. doi:10.1001/archpsyc.1990.01810150028006.

Fremont, Allen M., Paul D. Cleary, J. Lee Hargraves, Rachel M. Rowe, Nancy B. Jacobson, and John Z. Ayanian. 2001. "Patient-Centered

Processes Of Care And Long-Term Outcomes Of Myocardial Infarction." *Journal of General Internal Medicine* 16 (12): 800-808. doi:10.1046/j.1525-1497.2001.10102.x.

Fujisawa, Rie, and Nicolas S. Klazinga. 2017. "Measuring patient experiences (PREMS): Progress made by the OECD and its member countries between 2006 and 2016." *OECD Health Working Papers*, No. 102. https://doi.org/10.1787/893a07d2-en.

Gebhardt, Stefan, Anna Maria Wolak, and Martin Tobias Huber. 2013. "Patient Satisfaction And Clinical Parameters In Psychiatric Inpatients—The Prevailing Role Of Symptom Severity And Pharmacologic Disturbances." *Comprehensive Psychiatry* 54 (1): 53-60. doi:10.1016/j.comppsych.2012.03.016.

Gewandter, Jennifer S., S. Northwood, Maria Frazier, J. DelVecchio, S. Judge, C. Swanger, and John D. Markman. 2018. "A Prospective Study Of Patient Satisfaction With Communication Regarding Chronic Pain In The Primary Care Setting: Do Opioid Prescriptions Matter?" *The Journal of Pain* 19 (3): S55. doi:10.1016/j.jpain.2017.12.135.

Gignon, Maxime, Christine Ammirati, Romain Mercier, and Matthieu Detave. 2014. "Compliance With Emergency Department Discharge Instructions." *Journal of Emergency Nursing* 40 (1): 51-55. doi:10.1016/j.jen.2012.10.004.

Girotra, Saket, Peter Cram, and Ioana Popescu. 2012. "Patient Satisfaction At America's Lowest Performing Hospitals." *Circulation: Cardiovascular Quality and Outcomes* 5 (3): 365-372. doi:10.1161/circoutcomes.111.964361.

Glickman, Seth W., William Boulding, Matthew Manary, Richard Staelin, Matthew T. Roe, Robert J. Wolosin, E. Magnus Ohman, Eric D. Peterson, and Kevin A. Schulman. 2010. "Patient Satisfaction And Its Relationship With Clinical Quality And Inpatient Mortality In Acute Myocardial Infarction." *Circulation: Cardiovascular Quality And Outcomes* 3 (2): 188-195. doi:10.1161/circoutcomes.109.900597.

Glover, McKinley, Omid Khalilzadeh, Garry Choy, Anand M. Prabhakar, Pari V. Pandharipande, and G. Scott Gazelle. 2015. "Hospital Evaluations By Social Media: A Comparative Analysis Of Facebook

Ratings Among Performance Outliers." *Journal of General Internal Medicine* 30 (10): 1440-1446. doi:10.1007/s11606-015-3236-3.

Goldstein, Eric, Chuan-Xing Ho, Rania Hanna, Clara Elinger, Kathleen L. Yaremchuk, Michael D. Seidman, and Michelle T. Jesse. 2015. "Cost Of Care For Subjective Tinnitus In Relation To Patient Satisfaction." *Otolaryngology–Head and Neck Surgery* 152 (3): 518-523. doi:10.1177/0194599814566179.

Greenfield, Sheldon, Sherrie Kaplan, and John E. Ware. 1985. "Expanding Patient Involvement In Care." *Annals of Internal Medicine* 102 (4): 520. doi:10.7326/0003-4819-102-4-520.

Greenfield, Sheldon, Sherrie H. Kaplan, John E. Ware, Elizabeth Martin Yano, and Harrison J. L. Frank. 1988. "Patients' Participation In Medical Care." *Journal of General Internal Medicine* 3 (5): 448-457. doi:10.1007/bf02595921.

Gross, Revital, Hava Tabenkin, Avi Porath, Anthony Heymann, Miriam Greenstein, Boaz Porter, and Ronit Matzliach. 2003. "The Relationship Between Primary Care Physicians' Adherence To Guidelines For The Treatment Of Diabetes And Patient Satisfaction: Findings From A Pilot Study." *Family Practice* 20 (5): 563-569. doi:10.1093/fampra/cmg512.

Gupta, Digant, Christopher G. Lis, and Mark Rodeghier. 2013. "Can Patient Experience With Service Quality Predict Survival In Colorectal Cancer?" *Journal for Healthcare Quality* 35 (6): 37-43. doi:10.1111/j.1945-1474.2012.00217.x.

Gupta, Digant, Kamal Patel, and Christopher G. Lis. 2015. "Self-Rated Health Supersedes Patient Satisfaction With Service Quality As A Predictor Of Survival In Prostate Cancer." *Health and Quality of Life Outcomes* 13 (1). doi:10.1186/s12955-015-0334-1.

Gupta, Digant, Mark Rodeghier, and Christopher G. Lis. 2013. "Patient Satisfaction With Service Quality As A Predictor Of Survival Outcomes In Breast Cancer." *Supportive Care In Cancer* 22 (1): 129-134. doi:10.1007/s00520-013-1956-7.

Gupta, Digant, Mark Rodeghier, and Christopher. G. Lis. 2013. "Patient Satisfaction With Service Quality In An Oncology Setting:

Implications For Prognosis In Non-Small Cell Lung Cancer." *International Journal for Quality in Health Care* 25 (6): 696-703. doi:10.1093/intqhc/mzt070.

Gupta, Digant, Maurie Markman, Rodeghier, and Christopher Lis. 2012. "The Relationship Between Patient Satisfaction With Service Quality And Survival In Pancreatic Cancer." *Patient Preference and Adherence*, 765. doi:10.2147/ppa.s37900.

Hachem, Fadi, Jeff Canar, Francis Fullam, Andrew S. Gallan, Samuel Hohmann, and Catherine Johnson. 2014. "The Relationships Between HCAHPS Communication And Discharge Satisfaction Items And Hospital Readmissions." *Patient Experience Journal* 1 (2): 71-77. doi:10.35680/2372-0247.1022.

Hamilton, David. F., Judith V. Lane, Paul Gaston, James T. Patton, Dborah MacDonald, A. Hamish R. W. Simpson, and Colin R. Howie. 2013. "What Determines Patient Satisfaction With Surgery? A Prospective Cohort Study Of 4709 Patients Following Total Joint Replacement." *BMJ Open* 3 (4): e002525. doi:10.1136/bmjopen-2012-002525.

Harris, Matthew J., Brijesh Patel, and Simon Bowen. 2011. "Primary Care Access And Its Relationship With Emergency Department Utilisation: An Observational, Cross-Sectional, Ecological Study." *British Journal of General Practice* 61 (593): e787-e793. doi:10.3399/bjgp11x613124.

Heisler, Michele, Reynard R. Bouknight, Rodney A. Hayward, Dylan M. Smith, and Eve A. Kerr. 2002. "The Relative Importance Of Physician Communication, Participatory Decision Making, And Patient Understanding In Diabetes Self-Management." *Journal of General Internal Medicine* 17 (4): 243-252. doi:10.1046/j.1525-1497.2002.10905.x.

Helmerhorst, Gijs T. T., Anneluuk L. C. Lindenhovius, Mark Vrahas, David Ring, and Peter Kloen. 2012. "Satisfaction With Pain Relief After Operative Treatment Of An Ankle Fracture." *Injury* 43 (11): 1958-1961. doi:10.1016/j.injury.2012.08.018.

Henschke, Nicholas, Lara Wouda, Christopher G. Maher, Julia M. Hush, and Maurits W. van Tulder. 2013. "Determinants Of Patient Satisfaction 1 Year After Presenting To Primary Care With Acute Low

Back Pain." *The Clinical Journal of Pain* 29 (6): 512-517. doi:10.1097/ajp.0b013e318274b3e6.

Hodari, Kafele T., Jaleema R. Nanton, Christie L. Carroll, Steven R. Feldman, and Rajesh Balkrishnan. 2006. "Adherence In Dermatology: A Review Of The Last 20 Years." *Journal of Dermatological Treatment* 17 (3): 136-142. doi:10.1080/09546630600688515.

Hoff, Rani A., Robert A. Rosenheck, Mark Meterko, and Nancy J. Wilson. 1999. "Mental Illness As A Predictor Of Satisfaction With Inpatient Care At Veterans Affairs Hospitals." *Psychiatric Services* 50 (5): 680-685. doi:10.1176/ps.50.5.680.

Homma, Mieko, Hirono Ishikawa, and Takahiro Kiuchi. 2018. "Illness Perceptions And Negative Responses From Medical Professionals In Patients With Fibromyalgia: Association With Patient Satisfaction And Number Of Hospital Visits." *Patient Education and Counseling* 101 (3): 532-540. doi:10.1016/j.pec.2017.08.014.

Hoot, Nathan R., and Dominik Aronsky. 2008. "Systematic Review Of Emergency Department Crowding: Causes, Effects, And Solutions." *Annals of Emergency Medicine* 52 (2): 126-136.e1. doi:10.1016/j.annemergmed.2008.03.014.

Hopkins, Benjamin S., Mit R. Patel, Jonathan Tad Yamaguchi, Michael Brendan Cloney, and Nader S. Dahdaleh. 2019. "Predictors Of Patient Satisfaction And Survey Participation After Spine Surgery: A Retrospective Review Of 17,853 Consecutive Spinal Patients From A Single Academic Institution. Part 1: Press Ganey." *Journal of Neurosurgery: Spine* 30 (3): 382-388. doi:10.3171/2018.8.spine18594.

Hopkins, Benjamin S., Mit R. Patel, Jonathan Tad Yamaguchi, Michael Brendan Cloney, and Nader S. Dahdaleh. 2019. "Predictors Of Patient Satisfaction And Survey Participation After Spine Surgery: A Retrospective Review Of 17,853 Consecutive Spinal Patients From A Single Academic Institution. Part 2: HCAHPS." *Journal of Neurosurgery: Spine* 30 (3): 389-396. doi:10.3171/2018.8.spine181024.

Hussein, Mohamed G., Rehan Qayyam. 2015. "Abstract 12284: Hospital Patient Satisfaction Scores and 30-day Readmission and Mortality Rates of Heart Failure Patients." *Circulation* 132: A12284.

Husted, Henrik, Gitte Holm, and Steffen Jacobsen. 2008. "Predictors Of Length Of Stay And Patient Satisfaction After Hip And Knee Replacement Surgery: Fast-Track Experience In 712 Patients." *Acta Orthopaedica* 79 (2): 168-173. doi:10.1080/17453670710014941.

Hwang, Ula, Lynne D. Richardson, Tolulope O. Sonuyi, and R. Sean Morrison. 2006. "The Effect Of Emergency Department Crowding On The Management Of Pain In Older Adults With Hip Fracture." *Journal Of The American Geriatrics Society* 54 (2): 270-275. doi:10.1111/j.1532-5415.2005.00587.x.

Iannuzzi, James C., Steven A. Kahn, Linlin Zhang, Mark L. Gestring, Katia Noyes, and John R. T. Monson. 2015. "Getting Satisfaction: Drivers Of Surgical Hospital Consumer Assessment Of Health Care Providers And Systems Survey Scores." *Journal of Surgical Research* 197 (1): 155-161. doi:10.1016/j.jss.2015.03.045.

Institute of Medicine. *Crossing The Quality Chasm: A New Health System For The 21St Century*. 2001. Washington, D.C.: National Academy Press.

Isaac, Thomas, Alan M. Zaslavsky, Paul D. Cleary, and Bruce E. Landon. 2010. "The Relationship Between Patients' Perception Of Care And Measures Of Hospital Quality And Safety." *Health Services Research* 45 (4): 1024-1040. doi:10.1111/j.1475-6773.2010.01122.x.

Ismail, Sharif A., Daniel C. Gibbons, and Shamini Gnani. 2013. "Reducing Inappropriate Accident And Emergency Department Attendances:" *British Journal of General Practice* 63 (617): e813-e820. doi:10.3399/bjgp13x675395.

Jerant, Anthony, Alicia Agnoli, and Peter Franks. 2020. "Satisfaction With Health Care Among Prescription Opioid Recipients." *The Journal of The American Board of Family Medicine* 33 (1): 34-41. doi:10.3122/jabfm.2020.01.190090.

Jerant, Anthony, Kevin Fiscella, Joshua J. Fenton, Elizabeth M. Magnan, Alicia Agnoli, and Peter Franks. 2019. "Patient Satisfaction With

Clinicians And Short-Term Mortality In A US National Sample: The Roles Of Morbidity And Gender." *Journal of General Internal Medicine* 34 (8): 1459-1466. doi:10.1007/s11606-019-05058-8.

Jha, Ashish K., E. John Orav, Jie Zheng, and Arnold M. Epstein. 2008. "Patients' Perception Of Hospital Care In The United States." *New England Journal of Medicine* 359 (18): 1921-1931. doi:10.1056/nejmsa0804116.

Johnston, Emily M., Kenton J. Johnston, Jaeyong Bae, Jason M. Hockenberry, Arnold Milstein, and Edmund Becker. 2016. "Impact Of Hospital Diagnosis-Specific Quality Measures On Patients' Experience Of Hospital Care: Evidence From 14 States, 2009-2011." *Patient Experience Journal* 3 (1): 80-91. doi:10.35680/2372-0247.1128.

Jolly, Meenakshi, Bhavika Sethi, Courtney O'Brien, Winston Sequeira, Joel A. Block, Sergio Toloza, and Ana Bertoli et al. 2019. "Drivers Of Satisfaction With Care For Patients With Lupus." *ACR Open Rheumatology* 1 (10): 649-656. doi:10.1002/acr2.11085.

Joseph, Bellal, Asad Azim, Terence O'Keeffe, Kareem Ibraheem, Narong Kulvatunyou, Andrew Tang, Gary Vercruysse, Randall Friese, Rifat Latifi, and Peter Rhee. 2017. "American College Of Surgeons Level I Trauma Centers Outcomes Do Not Correlate With Patients' Perception Of Hospital Experience." *Journal of Trauma and Acute Care Surgery* 82 (4): 722-727. doi:10.1097/ta.0000000000001385.

Kavalnienė, Rima, Aušra Deksnyte, Vytautas Kasiulevičius, Virginijus Šapoka, Ramūnas Aranauskas, and Lukas Aranauskas. 2018. "Patient Satisfaction With Primary Healthcare Services: Are There Any Links With Patients' Symptoms Of Anxiety And Depression?" *BMC Family Practice* 19 (1). doi:10.1186/s12875-018-0780-z.

Kane, Robert L., Matthew Maciejewski, and Michael Finch. 1997. "The Relationship Of Patient Satisfaction With Care And Clinical Outcomes." *Medical Care* 35 (7): 714-730. doi:10.1097/00005650-199707000-00005.

Kaptain, George J., Nathan E. Simmons, Robert E. Replogle, and Louis Pobereskin. 2000. "Incidence And Outcome Of Kyphotic Deformity Following Laminectomy For Cervical Spondylotic Myelopathy."

Journal of Neurosurgery: Spine 93 (2): 199-204. doi:10.3171/spi.2000.93.2.0199.

Kelstrup, Anne Mette, Ketil Lund, B. Lauritsen, and Pascal Bech. 1993. "Satisfaction With Care Reported By Psychiatric Inpatients Relationship To Diagnosis And Medical Treatment." *Acta Psychiatrica Scandinavica* 87 (6): 374-379. doi:10.1111/j.1600-0447.1993.tb03390.x.

Kinnersley, Paul, Nigel Stott, Tim J. Peters, and Ian Harvey. 1999. "The patient-centredness of consultations and outcome in primary care." *The British Journal of General Practice: The Journal of the Royal College of General Practitioners* 49 (446): 711–716.

Kleeberg, Ulrich R., Jan-T.orsten Tews, Thomas M. Ruprecht, Mechtild Höing, Alexander Kuhlmann, and Clause Runge. 2005. "Patient Satisfaction And Quality Of Life In Cancer Outpatients: Results Of The PASQOC* Study." *Supportive Care In Cancer* 13 (5): 303-310. doi:10.1007/s00520-004-0727-x.

Köhler, Stephan, Theresa Unger, Sabine Hoffmann, Bruno Steinacher, and Thomas Fydrich. 2014. "Patient Satisfaction With Inpatient Psychiatric Treatment And Its Relation To Treatment Outcome In Unipolar Depression And Schizophrenia." *International Journal of Psychiatry in Clinical Practice* 19 (2): 119-123. doi:10.3109/13651501.2014.988272.

Kohring, Jessica M., Christopher E. Pelt, Mike B. Anderson, Christopher L. Peters, and Jeremy M. Gililland. 2018. "Press Ganey Outpatient Medical Practice Survey Scores Do Not Correlate With Patient-Reported Outcomes After Primary Joint Arthroplasty." *The Journal of Arthroplasty* 33 (8): 2417-2422. doi:10.1016/j.arth.2018.03.044.

Kondasani, Rama Koteswara Rao, and Rajeev Kumar Panda. 2015. "Customer Perceived Service Quality, Satisfaction And Loyalty In Indian Private Healthcare." *International Journal of Health Care Quality Assurance* 28 (5): 452-467. doi:10.1108/ijhcqa-01-2015-0008.

Korman, Neil J., Yang Zhao, Jakie Lu, and Mary Helen Tran. 2015. "Psoriasis disease severity affects patient satisfaction with treatment."

Dermatology Online Journal, 21(7). https://escholarship.org/uc/item/69h903m6.

Koulaxouzidis, Georgios, Arash Momeni, Filip Simunovic, Florian Lampert, Holger Bannasch, and G. Björn Stark. 2014. "Aesthetic Surgery Performed By Plastic Surgery Residents." *Annals of Plastic Surgery* 73 (6): 696-700. doi:10.1097/sap.0b013e31828d7090.

Kravitz, Richard L., Ronald M. Epstein, Mitchell D. Feldman, Carol E. Franz, Rahman Azari, Michael S. Wilkes, Ladson Hinton, and Peter Franks. 2005. "Influence Of Patients' Requests For Direct-To-Consumer Advertised Antidepressants." *JAMA* 293 (16): 1995. doi:10.1001/jama.293.16.1995.

Kronish, Ian M., Michael A. Diefenbach, Donald E. Edmondson, L. Alison Phillips, Kezhen Fei, and Carol R. Horowitz. 2013. "Key Barriers To Medication Adherence In Survivors Of Strokes And Transient Ischemic Attacks." *Journal of General Internal Medicine* 28 (5): 675-682. doi:10.1007/s11606-012-2308-x.

Lake, Eileen T., Hayley D. Germack, and Molly Kreider Viscardi. 2015. "Missed Nursing Care Is Linked To Patient Satisfaction: A Cross-Sectional Study Of US Hospitals." *BMJ Quality & Safety* 25 (7): 535-543. doi:10.1136/bmjqs-2015-003961.

Larson, Celia O., Eeguen C. Nelson, David Gustafson, and Paul B. Batalden. 1996. "The Relationship Between Meeting Patients' Information Needs And Their Satisfaction With Hospital Care And General Health Status Outcomes." *International Journal for Quality in Health Care* 8 (5): 447-456. doi:10.1093/intqhc/8.5.447.

Lee, Yin-Yang, and Julia L. Lin. 2010. "Do Patient Autonomy Preferences Matter? Linking Patient-Centered Care To Patient–Physician Relationships And Health Outcomes." *Social Science & Medicine* 71 (10): 1811-1818. doi:10.1016/j.socscimed.2010.08.008.

Levin, Jay M., Robert Winkelman, Gabriel A. Smith, Joseph E. Tanenbaum, Thomas E. Mroz, and Michael P. Steinmetz. 2017. "The Association Between The Hospital Consumer Assessment Of Healthcare Providers And Systems (HCAHPS) Survey And Real-

World Clinical Outcomes In Lumbar Spine Surgery." *The Spine Journal* 17 (10): S111-S112. doi:10.1016/j.spinee.2017.07.095.

Levinson, Wendy, Debra L. Roter, John P. Mullooly, Valerie T. Dull, and Richard M. Frankel. 1997. "Physician-Patient Communication. The Relationship With Malpractice Claims Among Primary Care Physicians And Surgeons." *JAMA* 277 (7): 553-559. doi:10.1001/jama.277.7.553.

Lewis, Eleanor T., Ann Combs, and Jodie A. Trafton. 2010. "Reasons For Under-Use Of Prescribed Opioid Medications By Patients In Pain." *Pain Medicine* 11 (6): 861-871. doi:10.1111/j.1526-4637.2010.00868.x.

Linetzky, Bruno, Dingfeng Jiang, Martha M. Funnell, Bradley H. Curtis, and William H. Polonsky. 2016. "Exploring The Role Of The Patient-Physician Relationship On Insulin Adherence And Clinical Outcomes In Type 2 Diabetes: Insights From The Mosaic Study." *Journal of Diabetes* 9 (6): 596-605. doi:10.1111/1753-0407.12443.

Li, Deborah J., Yikyung Park, Neeta Vachharajani, Wint Yan Aung, Jacqueline Garonzik-Wang, and William C. Chapman. 2017. "Physician-Patient Communication Is Associated With Hepatocellular Carcinoma Screening In Chronic Liver Disease Patients." *Journal of Clinical Gastroenterology* 51 (5): 454-460. doi:10.1097/mcg.0000000000000747.

Lis, Christopher G., Kamal Patel, and Digant Gupta. 2015. "The Relationship Between Patient Satisfaction With Service Quality And Survival In Non-Small Cell Lung Cancer – Is Self-Rated Health A Potential Confounder?" *PLOS ONE* 10 (7): e0134617. doi:10.1371/journal.pone.0134617.

Lis, Christopher G., Mark Rodeghier, and Digant Gupta. 2011. "The Relationship Between Perceived Service Quality And Patient Willingness To Recommend At A National Oncology Hospital Network." *BMC Health Services Research* 11 (1). doi:10.1186/1472-6963-11-46.

Lis, Christopher G., Mark Rodeghier, James F. Grutsch, and Digant Gupta. 2009. "Distribution And Determinants Of Patient Satisfaction In

Oncology With A Focus On Health Related Quality Of Life." *BMC Health Services Research* 9 (1). doi:10.1186/1472-6963-9-190.

Little, Paul, Hazel Everitt, Ian Williamson, Greg Warner, Michael Moore, Clare Gould, Kate Ferrier, and Shiela Payne. 2001. "Observational Study Of Effect Of Patient Centredness And Positive Approach On Outcomes Of General Practice Consultations." *BMJ* 323 (7318): 908-911. doi:10.1136/bmj.323.7318.908.

Liu, Jessica J., John Matelski, Peter Cram, David R. Urbach, and Chaim M. Bell. 2016. "Association Between Online Physician Ratings And Cardiac Surgery Mortality." *Circulation: Cardiovascular Quality and Outcomes* 9 (6): 788-791. doi:10.1161/circoutcomes.116.003016.

Llanwarne, Nadia R., Gary A. Abel, Marc N. Elliott, Charlotte A. M. Paddison, Georgios Lyratzopoulos, John L. Campbell, and Martin Roland. 2013. "Relationship Between Clinical Quality And Patient Experience: Analysis Of Data From The English Quality And Outcomes Framework And The National GP Patient Survey." *The Annals of Family Medicine* 11 (5): 467-472. doi:10.1370/afm.1514.

Lobo Prabhu, Kristel, Michelle C. Cleghorn, Ahmad Elnahas, Alvina Tse, Azusa Maeda, Fayez A. Quereshy, Allan Okrainec, and Timothy D. Jackson. 2017. "Is Quality Important To Our Patients? The Relationship Between Surgical Outcomes And Patient Satisfaction." *BMJ Quality & Safety* 27 (1): 48-52. doi:10.1136/bmjqs-2017-007071.

Lorish, Thomas R., Calvin T. Tanabe, Frederick T. Waller, Marla R. London, and David J. Lansky. 1998. "Correlation Between Health Outcome And Length Of Hospital Stay In Lumbar Microdiscectomy." *Spine* 23 (20): 2195-2200. doi:10.1097/00007632-199810150-00010.

Lyu, Heather, Michol Cooper, Julie A. Freischlag, and Martin A. Makary. 2013. "Patient Satisfaction As A Possible Indicator Of Quality Surgical Care—Reply." *JAMA Surgery* 148 (10): 986. doi:10.1001/jamasurg.2013.3411.

Macfarlane, John T., William Holmes, Rosamund Macfarlane, and Nicky Britten. 1997. "Influence Of Patients' Expectations On Antibiotic Management Of Acute Lower Respiratory Tract Illness In General

Practice: Questionnaire Study." *BMJ* 315 (7117): 1211-1214. doi:10.1136/bmj.315.7117.1211.

Maher, Dermot P., Pauline Woo, Waylan Wong, Xiao Zhang, Roya Yumul, and Charles Louy. 2016. "Perioperative Factors Associated With Hospital Consumer Assessment Of Healthcare Providers And Systems Responses Of Total Hip Arthroplasty Patients." *Journal of Clinical Anesthesia* 34: 232-238. doi:10.1016/j.jclinane.2016.03.047.

Male, Leanne, Adam Noble, Jessica Atkinson, and Tony Marson. 2017. "Measuring Patient Experience: A Systematic Review To Evaluate Psychometric Properties Of Patient Reported Experience Measures (Prems) For Emergency Care Service Provision." *International Journal For Quality In Health Care* 29 (3): 314-326. doi:10.1093/intqhc/mzx027.

Mancuso, Carol A., Eduardo A. Salvati, Norman A. Johanson, Margaret G. E. Peterson, and Mary E. Charlson. 1997. "Patients' Expectations And Satisfaction With Total Hip Arthroplasty." *The Journal of Arthroplasty* 12 (4): 387-396. doi:10.1016/s0883-5403(97)90194-7.

Mannion, Anne F., Francois Porchet, Frank S. Kleinstück, Friederike Lattig, Dezsoe Jeszenszky, Viktor Bartanusz, Jiri Dvorak, and Daniel Grob. 2009. "The Quality Of Spine Surgery From The Patient'S Perspective. Part 1: The Core Outcome Measures Index In Clinical Practice." *European Spine Journal* 18 (S3): 367-373. doi:10.1007/s00586-009-0942-8.

Martin, Alison, Christopher Martin, Peter B. Martin, Peter A. B. Martin, Gill Green, and Sandra Eldridge. 2002. "'Inappropriate' Attendance At An Accident And Emergency Department By Adults Registered In Local General Practices: How Is It Related To Their Use Of Primary Care?" *Journal of Health Services Research & Policy* 7 (3): 160-165. doi:10.1258/135581902760082463.

Mazurenko, Olena, Justin Blackburn, Matthew Bair, Areeba Kara, and Christopher A. Harle. 2019. "3038 Examining The Association Between Inpatient Opioid Prescribing And Patient Satisfaction." *Journal of Clinical and Translational Science* 3 (s1): 121-122. doi:10.1017/cts.2019.277.

McCracken, Lance M., Donna Evon, and Eleftheria T. Karapas. 2002. "Satisfaction With Treatment For Chronic Pain In A Specialty Service: Preliminary Prospective Results." *European Journal of Pain* 6 (5): 387-393. doi:10.1016/s1090-3801(02)00042-3.

McLean, Kenneth A., Z. Sheng, Stephen O'Neill, Kathryn Boyce, C. Jones, S.tephen J. Wigmore, and Ewen M. Harrison. 2017. "The Influence Of Clinical And Patient-Reported Outcomes On Post-Surgery Satisfaction In Cholecystectomy Patients." *World Journal of Surgery* 41 (7): 1752-1761. doi:10.1007/s00268-017-3917-7.

Mehta, Rittal, Diamantis I. Tsilimigras, Anghela Z. Paredes, Mary Dillhoff, Jordan M. Cloyd, Aslam Ejaz, Allan Tsung, and Timothy M. Pawlik. 2020. "Is Patient Satisfaction Dictated By Quality Of Care Among Patients Undergoing Complex Surgical Procedures For A Malignant Indication?" *Annals of Surgical Oncology*. doi:10.1245/s10434-020-08788-w.

Menendez, Joshua York, Nidal Bassam Omar, Gustavo Chagoya, Borna Ethan Tabibian, Galal Ashraf Elsayed, Beverly Claire Walters, Barton Lucius Guthrie, and Mark Norman Hadley. 2019. "Patient Satisfaction In Spine Surgery: A Systematic Review Of The Literature." *Asian Spine Journal* 13 (6): 1047-1057. doi:10.31616/asj.2019.0032.

Mesrobian, James, Sheila R. Barnett, Karen B. Dimino, David Mackey, Sonya Pease, and Richard Urman, 2020. *Patient Satisfaction With Anesthesia White Paper*. American Society of Anesthesiologists (ASA). Last modified 2020. https://www.asahq.org/quality-and-practice-management/quality-improvement/patient-satisfaction-with-anesthesia-white-paper.

Meterko, Mark, Steven Wright, Hai Lin, Elliott Lowy, and Paul D. Cleary. 2010. "Mortality Among Patients With Acute Myocardial Infarction: The Influences Of Patient-Centered Care And Evidence-Based Medicine." *Health Services Research* 45 (5p1): 1188-1204. doi:10.1111/j.1475-6773.2010.01138.x.

Mets, Elbert J., Michael R. Mercier, Ari S. Hilibrand, Michelle C. Scott, Arya G. Varthi, and Jonathan N. Grauer. 2020. "Patient-Related Factors And Perioperative Outcomes Are Associated With Self-

Reported Hospital Rating After Spine Surgery." *Clinical Orthopaedics and Related Research* 478 (3): 643-652. doi:10.1097/corr.0000000000000892.

Mills, Angela M., Frances S. Shofer, Esther H. Chen, Judd E. Hollander, and Jesse M. Pines. 2009. "The Association Between Emergency Department Crowding And Analgesia Administration In Acute Abdominal Pain Patients." *Academic Emergency Medicine* 16 (7): 603-608. doi:10.1111/j.1553-2712.2009.00441.x.

Mistry, Jaydev B., Chukwuweike U. Gwam, Morad Chughtai, Anton Khlopas, Prem Ramkumar, Nicolas S. Piuzzi, George Muschler, Steven F. Harwin, Michael A. Mont, and Ronald E. Delanois. 2017. "Factors Influencing Patients' Hospital Rating After Total Joint Arthroplasty." *Orthopedics* 40 (6): 377-380. doi:10.3928/01477447-20171019-03.

Mistry, Jaydev B., Morad Chughtai, Randa K. Elmallah, Sidney Le, Peter M. Bonutti, Ronald E. Delanois, and Michael A. Mont. 2016. "What Influences How Patients Rate Their Hospital After Total Hip Arthroplasty?." *The Journal Arthroplasty* 31 (11): 2422-2425. doi:10.1016/j.arth.2016.03.060.

Mohamed, Nequesha S., Chukwuweike U. Gwam, Jennifer I. Etcheson, Iciar M. Dávila Castrodad, Steven L. Gitarts, Avnish S. Jetty, Brandon A. Srour, and Ronald E. Delanois. 2018. "Pain Intensity: How Press Ganey Survey Domains Correlate In Total Knee Arthroplasty Patients." *The Journal of Knee Surgery* 33 (01): 048-052. doi:10.1055/s-0038-1676517.

Mold, James W., George E. Fryer, and A. Michelle Roberts. 2004. "When Do Older Patients Change Primary Care Physicians?" *The Journal of The American Board of Family Medicine* 17 (6): 453-460. doi:10.3122/jabfm.17.6.453.

Molfenter, Todd D., and Roger Brown. 2014. "Effects Of Physician Communication And Family Hardiness On Patient Medication Regimen Beliefs And Adherence." *General Medicine: Open Access* 02 (03). doi:10.4172/2327-5146.1000136.

Müller, Ophélie, Cédric Baumann, Paolo Di Patrizio, Sarah Viennet, Guillaume Vlamynck, Laura Collet, Isabelle Clerc-Urmès, Raymund Schwan, and Stéphanie Bourion-Bédès. 2020. "Patient's Early Satisfaction With Care: A Predictor Of Health-Related Quality Of Life Change Among Outpatients With Substance Dependence." *Health And Quality Of Life Outcomes* 18 (1). doi:10.1186/s12955-019-1267-x.

Myles, Paul S., Darryl L. Williams, Melisa Hendrata, Hugh Anderson, and A nthony M. Weeks. 2000. "Patient Satisfaction After Anaesthesia And Surgery: Results Of A Prospective Survey Of 10,811 Patients." *British Journal of Anaesthesia* 84 (1): 6-10. doi:10.1093/oxfordjournals.bja.a013383.

Nagraj, Shobhana, Gary Abel, Charlotte Paddison, Rupert Payne, Marc Elliott, John Campbell, and Martin Roland. 2013. "Changing Practice As A Quality Indicator For Primary Care: Analysis Of Data On Voluntary Disenrollment From The English GP Patient Survey." *BMC Family Practice* 14 (1). doi:10.1186/1471-2296-14-89.

Nalliah, Romesh P., Kenneth R. Sloss, Brooke C. Kenney, Sarah K. Bettag, Shernel Thomas, Kendall Dubois, Jennifer F. Waljee, and Chad M. Brummett. 2020. "Association Of Opioid Use With Pain And Satisfaction After Dental Extraction." *JAMA Network Open* 3 (3): e200901. doi:10.1001/jamanetworkopen.2020.0901.

Narayan, K. M. Venkat, Edward W. Gregg, Anne Fagot-Campagna, Tiffany L. Gary, Jinan B. Saaddine, Corette Parker, Giuseppina Imperatore, Rodolfo Valdez, Gloria Beckles, and Michael M. Engelgau. 2003. "Relationship between quality of diabetes care and patient satisfaction." *Journal of the National Medical Association* 95 (1): 64–70.

Nasir, Nik M., Franzza Ariffin, and Siti Munira. 2018. "Physician-patient interaction satisfaction and its influence on medication adherence and type-2 diabetic control in a primary care setting." *The Medical journal of Malaysia* 73 (3): 163–169.

Nasir, Khurram, and Victor Okunrintemi. 2018. "Association Of Patient-Reported Experiences With Health Resource Utilization And Cost Among US Adult Population, Medical Expenditure Panel Survey

(MEPS), 2010–13." *International Journal for Quality in Health Care* 31 (7): 547-555. doi:10.1093/intqhc/mzy217.

Nassiri, Ashley M., Scott J. Stephan, Liping Du, William R. Ries, and Roland D. Eavey. 2020. "Factors Associated With Patient Satisfaction After Nasal Breathing Surgery." *JAMA Network Open* 3 (3): e201409. doi:10.1001/jamanetworkopen.2020.1409.

National Institute for Health and Care Excellence. 2012. *Patient experience in adult NHS services.* Last modified July 31, 2019. https://www.nice.org.uk/guidance/qs15/chapter/Quality-statements.

Neri, Luca, Ketty Peris, Caterina Longo, Stefano Calvieri, Pasquale Frascione, Aurora Parodi, and Laura Eibenschuz et al. 2018. "Physician–Patient Communication And Patient-Reported Outcomes In The Actinic Keratosis Treatment Adherence Initiative (AK - TRAIN): A Multicenter, Prospective, Real-Life Study Of Treatment Satisfaction, Quality Of Life And Adherence To Topical Field-Directed Therapy For The Treatment Of Actinic Keratosis In Italy." *Journal of The European Academy of Dermatology And Venereology* 33 (1): 93-107. doi:10.1111/jdv.15142.

Newton, Peter O., Vidyadhar V. Upasani, Tracey P. Bastrom, and Michelle C. Marks. 2009. "The Deformity-Flexibility Quotient Predicts Both Patient Satisfaction And Surgeon Preference In The Treatment Of Lenke 1B Or 1C Curves For Adolescent Idiopathic Scoliosis." *Spine* 34 (10): 1032-1039. doi:10.1097/brs.0b013e31819c97f8.

Nicoloro-SantaBarbara, Jennifer, Lisa Rosenthal, Melissa V. Auerbach, Christina Kocis, Cheyanne Busso, and Marci Lobel. 2017. "Patient-Provider Communication, Maternal Anxiety, And Self-Care In Pregnancy." *Social Science & Medicine* 190: 133-140. doi:10.1016/j.socscimed.2017.08.011.

North, Frederick, Sarah J. Crane, Jon O. Ebbert, and Sidna M. Tulledge-Scheitel. 2018. "Do Primary Care Providers Who Prescribe More Opioids Have Higher Patient Panel Satisfaction Scores?" *SAGE Open Medicine* 6: 205031211878254. doi:10.1177/2050312118782547.

Nota, Sjoerd P. F. T., Silke A. Spit, Timothy Voskuyl, Arjan G. J. Bot, Michiel G. J. S. Hageman, and David Ring. 2015. "Opioid Use,

Satisfaction, And Pain Intensity After Orthopedic Surgery." *Psychosomatics* 56 (5): 479-485. doi:10.1016/j.psym.2014.09.003.

O'Brien, Marlene T., James C. Iannuzzi, Steven A. Kahn, Mark L. Gestring, John R. Monson, and David L. Gillespie. 2013. "Factors Associated With HCAHPS Performance In Vascular Surgery Patients." *Journal of Vascular Surgery* 57 (5): 95S-96S. doi:10.1016/j.jvs.2013.02.223.

Oetzel, John, Bryan Wilcox, Magdalena Avila, Ricky Hill, Ashley Archiopoli, and Tamar Ginossar. 2015. "Patient–Provider Interaction, Patient Satisfaction, And Health Outcomes: Testing Explanatory Models For People Living With HIV/AIDS." *AIDS Care* 27 (8): 972-978. doi:10.1080/09540121.2015.1015478.

Olivero, William C., Dorla Vinson, Charles Pierce, and Sarah Trumbull. 2017. "106 Correlation Between Press Ganey Scores And Quality Outcomes From N2QOD (Lumbar Spine) For A Hospital Employed Neurosurgical Practice." *Neurosurgery* 64 (CN_suppl_1): 221-221. doi:10.1093/neuros/nyx417.106.

Okunrintemi, Victor, Erica S. Spatz, Paul Di Capua, Joseph A. Salami, Javier Valero-Elizondo, Haider Warraich, and Salim S. Virani et al. 2017. "Patient–Provider Communication And Health Outcomes Among Individuals With Atherosclerotic Cardiovascular Disease In The United States." *Circulation: Cardiovascular Quality and Outcomes* 10 (4). doi:10.1161/circoutcomes.117.003635.

O'Malley, Ann S. 2013. "After-Hours Access To Primary Care Practices Linked With Lower Emergency Department Use And Less Unmet Medical Need." *Health Affairs* 32 (1): 175-183. doi:10.1377/hlthaff.2012.0494.

Patel, Nirav K., Eric Kim, Anton Khlopas, Morad Chughtai, Chukwuweike Gwam, Randa K. Elmallah, Prem Ramkumar, Nicholas S. Piuzzi, Ronald E. Delanois, George Muschler, and Michael A. Mont. 2017. "What Influences How Patients Rate Their Hospital Stay After Total Hip Arthroplasty?" *Surgical Technology International 30*: 405–410.

Peláez, Sandra, Alexandrine J. Lamontagne, Johanne Collin, Annie Gauthier, Roland M. Grad, Lucie Blais, and Kim L. Lavoie et al. 2015.

"Patients' Perspective Of Barriers And Facilitators To Taking Long-Term Controller Medication For Asthma: A Novel Taxonomy." *BMC Pulmonary Medicine* 15 (1). doi:10.1186/s12890-015-0044-9.

Perez, Victoria, and Seth Freedman. 2018. "Do Crowdsourced Hospital Ratings Coincide With Hospital Compare Measures Of Clinical And Nonclinical Quality?" *Health Services Research* 53 (6): 4491-4506. doi:10.1111/1475-6773.13026.

Peterson, Emily B., Jamie S. Ostroff, Katherine N. DuHamel, Thomas A. D'Agostino, Marisol Hernandez, Mollie R. Canzona, and Carma L. Bylund. 2016. "Impact Of Provider-Patient Communication On Cancer Screening Adherence: A Systematic Review." *Preventive Medicine* 93: 96-105. doi:10.1016/j.ypmed.2016.09.034.

Pham, Hoangmai H., Bruce E. Landon, James D. Reschovsky, Beny Wu, and Deborah Schrag. 2009. "Rapidity And Modality Of Imaging For Acute Low Back Pain In Elderly Patients." *Archives of Internal Medicine* 169 (10): 972. doi:10.1001/archinternmed.2009.78.

Pines, Jesse M., A. Russell Localio, Judd E. Hollander, William G. Baxt, Hoi Lee, Carolyn Phillips, and Joshua P. Metlay. 2007. "The Impact Of Emergency Department Crowding Measures On Time To Antibiotics For Patients With Community-Acquired Pneumonia." *Annals of Emergency Medicine* 50 (5): 510-516. doi:10.1016/j.annemergmed.2007.07.021.

Pines, Jesse M., Charles V. Pollack, Deborah B. Diercks, Anna Marie Chang, Frances S. Shofer, and Judd E. Hollander. 2009. "The Association Between Emergency Department Crowding And Adverse Cardiovascular Outcomes In Patients With Chest Pain." *Academic Emergency Medicine* 16 (7): 617-625. doi:10.1111/j.1553-2712.2009.00456.x.

Pines, Jesse M., and Judd E. Hollander. 2008. "Emergency Department Crowding Is Associated With Poor Care For Patients With Severe Pain." *Annals of Emergency Medicine* 51 (1): 1-5. doi:10.1016/j.annemergmed.2007.07.008.

Pines, Jesse M., Frances S. Shofer, Joshua A. Isserman, Stephanie B. Abbuhl, and Angela M. Mills. 2010. "The Effect Of Emergency

Department Crowding On Analgesia In Patients With Back Pain In Two Hospitals." *Academic Emergency Medicine* 17 (3): 276-283. doi:10.1111/j.1553-2712.2009.00676.x.

Plomondon, Mary E., David J. Magid, Frederick A. Masoudi, Philip G. Jones, Lisa C. Barry, Edward Havranek, Eric D. Peterson, Harlan M. Krumholz, John A. Spertus, and John S. Rumsfeld. 2007. "Association Between Angina And Treatment Satisfaction After Myocardial Infarction." *Journal of General Internal Medicine* 23 (1): 1-6. doi:10.1007/s11606-007-0430-y.

Plunkett, Patrick K., Declan G. Byrne, Tomás Breslin, Kathleen Bennett, and Bernard Silke. 2011. "Increasing Wait Times Predict Increasing Mortality For Emergency Medical Admissions." *European Journal of Emergency Medicine* 18 (4): 192-196. doi:10.1097/mej.0b013e328344917e.

Pound, Pandora, Kate Tilling, Anthony G. Rudd, and Charles D. A. Wolfe. 1999. "Does Patient Satisfaction Reflect Differences In Care Received After Stroke?" *Stroke* 30 (1): 49-55. doi:10.1161/01.str.30.1.49.

Pozdnyakova, Anastasia, Avery Tung, Richard Dutton, Anum Wazir, and David B. Glick. 2019. "Factors Affecting Patient Satisfaction With Their Anesthesiologist." *Anesthesia & Analgesia* 129 (4): 951-959. doi:10.1213/ane.0000000000004256.

Press Ganey. 2020. *Press Ganey Associates.* Accessed July 11, 2020. https://www.pressganey.com/.

Rabeneck, Linda, Kimberly Wristers, Julie Souchek, Terri Menke, Eunice Ambriz, and Nelda Wray. 2000. "Patient Satisfaction In Dyspepsia Is Related To Pain Symptoms." *Gastroenterology* 118 (4): A216. doi:10.1016/s0016-5085(00)82939-x.

Rai, Ashish, Xuesong Han, Zhiyuan Zheng, K. Robin Yabroff, and Ahmedin Jemal. 2018. "Determinants And Outcomes Of Satisfaction With Healthcare Provider Communication Among Cancer Survivors." *Journal of The National Comprehensive Cancer Network* 16 (8): 975-984. doi:10.6004/jnccn.2018.7034.

RAND Healthcare. 2020. *Patient Satisfaction Questionnaire.* Accessed July 11, 2020. https://www.rand.org/health-care/surveys_tools/psq.html.

Rao, Mala, Aileen Clarke, Colin Sanderson, and Richard Hammersley. 2006. "Patients' Own Assessments Of Quality Of Primary Care Compared With Objective Records Based Measures Of Technical Quality of Care: Cross Sectional Study." *BMJ* 333 (7557): 19. doi:10.1136/bmj.38874.499167.7c.

Ren, Xinhua S., Lewis Kazis, Austin Lee, William Rogers, and Susan Pendergrass. 2001. "Health Status And Satisfaction With Health Care: A Longitudinal Study Among Patients Served By The Veterans Health Administration." *American Journal of Medical Quality* 16 (5): 166-173. doi:10.1177/106286060101600504.

Reponen, Elina, Hanna Tuominen, Juha Hernesniemi, and Miikka Korja. 2015. "Patient Satisfaction And Short-Term Outcome In Elective Cranial Neurosurgery." *Neurosurgery* 77 (5): 769-776. doi:10.1227/neu.0000000000000931.

Richards, Helen L., Donal G. Fortune, and Christopher E. M. Griffiths. 2006. "Adherence To Treatment In Patients With Psoriasis." *Journal Of The European Academy of Dermatology and Venereology* 20 (4): 370-379. doi:10.1111/j.1468-3083.2006.01565.x.

Richardson, Drew B. 2006. "Increase In Patient Mortality At 10 Days Associated With Emergency Department Overcrowding." *Medical Journal of Australia* 184 (5): 213-216. doi:10.5694/j.1326-5377.2006.tb00204.x.

Rodriguez, Hector P., Angie Mae C. Rodday, Richard E. Marshall, Kimberly L. Nelson, William H. Rogers, and Dana G. Safran. 2007. "Relation Of Patients' Experiences With Individual Physicians To Malpractice Risk." *International Journal for Quality In Health Care* 20 (1): 5-12. doi:10.1093/intqhc/mzm065.

Rogers, Frederick, Michael Horst, Tuc To, Amelia Rogers, Mathew Edavettal, Daniel Wu, Jeffrey Anderson, John Lee, Turner Osler, and Lisa Brosey. 2013. "Factors Associated With Patient Satisfaction Scores For Physician Care In Trauma Patients." *Journal of Trauma*

And Acute Care Surgery 75 (1): 110-115. doi:10.1097/ta.0b013e318298484f.

Rostami, Mina, Leila Ahmadian, Yunes Jahani, and Aliakbar Niknafs. 2018. "The Effect Of Patient Satisfaction With Academic Hospitals On Their Loyalty." *The International Journal of Health Planning and Management* 34 (1). doi:10.1002/hpm.2685.

Rubin, Haya R., Barbara Gandek, William H. Rogers, Mark Kosinski, Colleen A. McHorney, and John E. Ware. 1993. "Patients' Ratings Of Outpatient Visits In Different Practice Settings." *JAMA* 270 (7): 835. doi:10.1001/jama.1993.03510070057036.

Rust, George, Jiali Ye, Peter Baltrus, Elvan Daniels, Barnidele Adesunloye, and George E. Fryer. 2008. "Practical Barriers To Timely Primary Care Access." *Archives of Internal Medicine* 168 (15): 1705. doi:10.1001/archinte.168.15.1705.

Sacks, Greg D., Elise H. Lawson, Aaron J. Dawes, Marcia M. Russell, Melinda Maggard-Gibbons, David S. Zingmond, and Clifford Y. Ko. 2015. "Relationship Between Hospital Performance On A Patient Satisfaction Survey And Surgical Quality." *JAMA Surgery* 150 (9): 858. doi:10.1001/jamasurg.2015.1108.

Safran Dana G., Jana E. Montgomery, Hong Chang, Julia Murphy, and William H. Rogers. 2001. "Switching doctors: predictors of voluntary disenrollment from a primary physician's practice." *Journal of Family Practice* 50 (2): 130-136.

Säilä, Tiina, Elina Mattila, Minna Kaila, Pirjo Aalto, and Marja Kaunonen. 2008. "Measuring Patient Assessments Of The Quality Of Outpatient Care: A Systematic Review." *Journal of Evaluation in Clinical Practice* 14 (1): 148-154. doi:10.1111/j.1365-2753.2007.00824.x.

Schmocker, Ryan K., Linda M. Cherney Stafford, and Emily R. Winslow. 2019. "Satisfaction With Surgeon Care As Measured By The Surgery-CAHPS Survey Is Not Related To NSQIP Outcomes." *Surgery* 165 (3): 510-515. doi:10.1016/j.surg.2018.08.028.

Schneider, Eric C., Alan M. Zaslavsky, Bruce E. Landon, Terry R. Lied, Stephen Sheingold, and Paul D. Cleary. 2001. "National Quality

Monitoring Of Medicare Health Plans." *Medical Care* 39 (12): 1313-1325. doi:10.1097/00005650-200112000-00007.

Schiffman, Michael, Salvador A. Brau, Robin Henderson, and Gwen Gimmestad. 2003. "Bilateral Implantation Of Low-Profile Interbody Fusion Cages: Subsidence, Lordosis, And Fusion Analysis." *The Spine Journal* 3 (5): 377-387. doi:10.1016/s1529-9430(03)00145-1.

Schoenfelder, Tonio, Joerg Klewer, and Joachim Kugler. 2011. "Analysis Of Factors Associated With Patient Satisfaction In Ophthalmology: The Influence Of Demographic Data, Visit Characteristics And Perceptions Of Received Care." *Ophthalmic and Physiological Optics* 31 (6): 580-587. doi:10.1111/j.1475-1313.2011.00869.x.

Schoenthaler, Antoinette M., Brian S. Schwartz, Craig Wood, and Walter F. Stewart. 2012. "Patient And Physician Factors Associated With Adherence To Diabetes Medications." *The Diabetes Educator* 38 (3): 397-408. doi:10.1177/0145721712440333.

Schoenthaler, Antoinette, William F. Chaplin, John P. Allegrante, Senaida Fernandez, Marleny Diaz-Gloster, Jonathan N. Tobin, and Gbenga Ogedegbe. 2009. "Provider Communication Effects Medication Adherence In Hypertensive African Americans." *Patient Education and Counseling* 75 (2): 185-191. doi:10.1016/j.pec.2008.09.018.

Schull, Michael J., Marian Vermeulen, Graham Slaughter, Laurie Morrison, and Paul Daly. 2004. "Emergency Department Crowding And Thrombolysis Delays In Acute Myocardial Infarction." *Annals of Emergency Medicine* 44 (6): 577-585. doi:10.1016/j.annemergmed.2004.05.004.

Schwartz, Tayler M., Miao Tai, Kavita M. Babu, and Roland C. Merchant. 2014. "Lack Of Association Between Press Ganey Emergency Department Patient Satisfaction Scores And Emergency Department Administration Of Analgesic Medications." *Annals of Emergency Medicine* 64 (5): 469-481. doi:10.1016/j.annemergmed.2014.02.010.

Sequist, Thomas D., Eric C. Schneider, Michael Anastario, Esosa G. Odigie, Richard Marshall, William H. Rogers, and Dana Gelb Safran. 2008. "Quality Monitoring Of Physicians: Linking Patients' Experiences Of Care To Clinical Quality And Outcomes." *Journal of*

General Internal Medicine 23 (11): 1784-1790. doi:10.1007/s11606-008-0760-4.

Serber, Eva R., Terry A. Cronan, and Heather R. Walen. 2003. "Predictors Of Patient Satisfaction And Health Care Costs For Patients With Fibromyalgia." *Psychology & Health* 18 (6): 771-787. doi:10.1080/0887044031000148237.

Shapiro, Robyn S., Deborah E. Simpson, Steven L. Lawrence, Anne Marie Talsky, Kathleen A. Sobocinski, and David L. Schiedermayer. 1989. "A Survey Of Sued And Nonsued Physicians And Suing Patients." *Archives of Internal Medicine* 149 (10): 2190-2196. doi:10.1001/archinte.149.10.2190.

Sharp, Adam L., Ernest Shen, Yi-Lin Wu, Adeline Wong, Michael Menchine, Michael H. Kanter, and Michael K. Gould. 2018. "Satisfaction with care after reducing opioids for chronic pain." *The American Journal of Managed Care* 24 (6): e196–e199.

Sheetz, Kyle H., Seth A. Waits, Micah E. Girotti, Darrell A. Campbell, and Michael J. Englesbe. 2014. "Patients' Perspectives Of Care And Surgical Outcomes In Michigan." *Annals of Surgery* 260 (1): 5-9. doi:10.1097/sla.0000000000000626.

Shirk, Joseph D., Hung-Jui Tan, Jim C. Hu, Christopher S. Saigal, and Mark S. Litwin. 2016. "Patient Experience And Quality Of Urologic Cancer Surgery In US Hospitals." *Cancer* 122 (16): 2571-2578. doi:10.1002/cncr.30081.

Siddiqui, Zishan, Stephen Berry, Amanda Bertram, Lisa Allen, Erik Hoyer, Nowella Durkin, Rehan Qayyum, Elizabeth Wick, Peter Pronovost, and Daniel J. Brotman. 2018. "Does Patient Experience Predict 30-Day Readmission? A Patient-Level Analysis Of HCAHPS Data." *Journal of Hospital Medicine* 13 (10): 681-687. doi:10.12788/jhm.3037.

Singer, Emily S., Robert E. Merritt, Desmond M. D'Souza, Susan D. Moffatt-Bruce, and Peter J. Kneuertz. 2019. "Patient Satisfaction After Lung Cancer Surgery: Do Clinical Outcomes Affect Hospital Consumer Assessment Of Health Care Providers And Systems Scores?" *The Annals of Thoracic Surgery* 108 (6): 1656-1663. doi:10.1016/j.athoracsur.2019.06.080.

Sites, Brian D., Jordon Harrison, Michael D. Herrick, Melissa M. Masaracchia, Michael L. Beach, and Matthew A. Davis. 2018. "Prescription Opioid Use And Satisfaction With Care Among Adults With Musculoskeletal Conditions." *The Annals of Family Medicine* 16 (1): 6-13. doi:10.1370/afm.2148.

Smith, Gabriel A., Steven Chirieleison, Jay Levin, Karam Atli, Robert Winkelman, Joseph E. Tanenbaum, Thomas Mroz, and Michael Steinmetz. 2019. "Impact Of Length Of Stay On HCAHPS Scores Following Lumbar Spine Surgery." *Journal Of Neurosurgery: Spine* 31 (3): 366-371. doi:10.3171/2019.3.spine181180.

Solberg, Leif I., Stephen E. Asche, Beth M. Averbeck, Anita M. Hayek, Kay G. Schmitt, Tim C. Lindquist, and Richard R. Carlson. 2008. "Can Patient Safety Be Measured By Surveys Of Patient Experiences?" *The Joint Commission Journal on Quality and Patient Safety* 34 (5): 266-274. doi:10.1016/s1553-7250(08)34033-1.

Soljak, Michael, Amaia Calderon-Larrañaga, Pankaj Sharma, Elizabeth Cecil, Derek Bell, Gerrard Abi-Aad, and Azeem Majeed. 2011. "Does Higher Quality Primary Health Care Reduce Stroke Admissions? A National Cross-Sectional Study." *British Journal of General Practice* 61 (593): e801-e807. doi:10.3399/bjgp11x613142.

Sox, Harold C., Iris Margulies, and Carol H. Sox. 1981. "Psychologically Mediated Effects Of Diagnostic Tests." *Annals Of Internal Medicine* 95 (6): 680. doi:10.7326/0003-4819-95-6-680.

Sprivulis, Peter C., Julie-Ann Da Silva, Ian G. Jacobs, Amanda R. L. Frazer, and George A. Jelinek. 2006. "The Association Between Hospital Overcrowding And Mortality Among Patients Admitted Via Western Australian Emergency Departments." *Medical Journal of Australia* 184 (12): 616-616. doi:10.5694/j.1326-5377.2006.tb00416.x.

Stamp, Kelly D., Jane Flanagan, Matt Gregas, and Judith Shindul-Rothschild. 2014. "Predictors Of Excess Heart Failure Readmissions." *Journal of Nursing Care Quality* 29 (2): 115-123. doi:10.1097/ncq.0000000000000042.

Stavropoulou, Charitini. 2011. "Non-Adherence To Medication And Doctor–Patient Relationship: Evidence From A European Survey."

Patient Education And Counseling 83 (1): 7-13. doi:10.1016/j.pec.2010.04.039.

Stein, Murray B., Peter P. Roy-Byrne, Michelle G. Craske, Laura Campbell-Sills, Ariel J. Lang, Daniella Golinelli, Raphael D. Rose, Alexander Bystritsky, Greer Sullivan, and Cathy D. Sherbourne. 2011. "Quality Of And Patient Satisfaction With Primary Health Care For Anxiety Disorders." *The Journal of Clinical Psychiatry* 72 (07): 970-976. doi:10.4088/jcp.09m05626blu.

Stewart, Moira A. 1995. "Effective physician-patient communication and health outcomes: a review." *Canadian Medical Association Journal* 152 (9): 1423-1433.

Stewart, Moira, Judith B. Brown, Alan Donner, Ian R. McWhinney, Julian Oates, Way W. Weston, and John Jordan. 2000. "The impact of patient-centered care on outcomes." *The Journal of Family Practice*, 49(9), 796–804.

Suhonen, Riitta, Minna Stolt, Agneta Berg, Jouko Katajisto, Chryssoula Lemonidou, Elisabeth Patiraki, Katarina Sjövall, and Andreas Charalambous. 2017. "Cancer Patients' Perceptions Of Quality-Of-Care Attributes-Associations With Age, Perceived Health Status, Gender And Education." *Journal of Clinical Nursing* 27 (1-2): 306-316. doi:10.1111/jocn.13902.

Sutcliffe, Nurhan, Ann E. Clarke, R Taylor, C Frost, and David A. Isenberg. 2001. "Total Costs And Predictors Of Costs In Patients With Systemic Lupus Erythematosus." *Rheumatology* 40 (1): 37-47. doi:10.1093/rheumatology/40.1.37.

Tashjian, Robert Z., Michael P. Bradley, Stephen Tocci, Jesus Rey, Ralph F. Henn, and Andrew Green. 2007. "Factors Influencing Patient Satisfaction After Rotator Cuff Repair." *Journal Of Shoulder And Elbow Surgery* 16 (6): 752-758. doi:10.1016/j.jse.2007.02.136.

Tevis, Sarah E., Gregory D. Kennedy, and K. Craig Kent. 2015. "Is There A Relationship Between Patient Satisfaction And Favorable Surgical Outcomes?" *Advances in Surgery* 49 (1): 221-233. doi:10.1016/j.yasu.2015.03.006.

The Beryl Institute. 2020. "Defining Patient Experience." Accessed July 11, 2020. https://www.theberylinstitute.org/page/DefiningPX.

Thoma-Perry, Carly, Ethan Charles Blocher-Smith, Lewis Jacobsen, and Jonathan Saxe. 2018. "HCAHPS Scores As A Surrogate For Quality Does Not Correlate With TQIP Quality Measures At A Level 1 Trauma Center." *Surgery* 164 (4): 810-813. doi:10.1016/j.surg.2018.07.032.

Thomas, Eric J., Helen R. Burstin, Anne C. O'Neil, E. John Orav, and Troyen A. Brennan. 1996. "Patient Noncompliance With Medical Advice After The Emergency Department Visit." *Annals Of Emergency Medicine* 27 (1): 49-55. doi:10.1016/s0196-0644(96)70296-2.

Thorneloe, Rachael J., Chris Bundy, Christopher E. M. Griffiths, Darren M. Ashcroft, and Lis Cordingley. 2012. "Adherence To Medication In Patients With Psoriasis: A Systematic Literature Review." *British Journal of Dermatology* 168 (1): 20-31. doi:10.1111/bjd.12039.

Timian, Alex, Sonia Rupcic, Stan Kachnowski, and Paloma Luisi. 2013. "Do Patients "Like" Good Care? Measuring Hospital Quality Via Facebook." *American Journal of Medical Quality* 28 (5): 374-382. doi:10.1177/1062860612474839.

Tsai, Thomas C., E. John Orav, and Ashish K. Jha. 2015. "Patient Satisfaction And Quality Of Surgical Care In US Hospitals." *Annals of Surgery* 261 (1): 2-8. doi:10.1097/sla.0000000000000765.

van den Berg, Michael J, Tessa van Loenen, and Gert P. Westert. 2015. "Accessible And Continuous Primary Care May Help Reduce Rates Of Emergency Department Use. An International Survey In 34 Countries." *Family Practice* 33 (1): 42-50. doi:10.1093/fampra/cmv082.

Viccellio, Asa, Carolyn Santora, Adam J. Singer, Henry C. Thode, and Mark C. Henry. 2009. "The Association Between Transfer Of Emergency Department Boarders To Inpatient Hallways And Mortality: A 4-Year Experience." *Annals of Emergency Medicine* 54 (4): 487-491. doi:10.1016/j.annemergmed.2009.03.005.

Vincent, Charles. 2003. "Understanding And Responding To Adverse Events." *New England Journal of Medicine* 348 (11): 1051-1056. doi:10.1056/nejmhpr020760.

Waljee, Jennifer F., Emily S. Hu, Lisa A. Newman, and Amy K. Alderman. 2008. "Correlates Of Patient Satisfaction And Provider Trust After Breast-Conserving Surgery." *Cancer* 112 (8): 1679-1687. doi:10.1002/cncr.23351.

Wang, Hsiu-Ling, Jun-Ying Huang, and Shen-Long Howng. 2011. "The Effect On Patient Loyalty Of Service Quality, Patient Visit Experience And Perceived Switching Costs: Lessons From One Taiwan University Hospital." *Health Services Management Research* 24 (1): 29-36. doi:10.1258/hsmr.2010.010011.

Ward, Michael M., Saigeetha Sundaramurthy, Debra Lotstein, Thomas M. Bush, C. Michael Neuwelt, and Richard L. Street. 2003. "Participatory Patient-Physician Communication And Morbidity In Patients With Systemic Lupus Erythematosus." *Arthritis & Rheumatism* 49 (6): 810-818. doi:10.1002/art.11467.

Ware, John E., Allyson R. Davies-Avery, and Anita L Stewart. 1978. "The measurement and meaning of patient satisfaction." *Health & Medical Care Services Review* 1 (1): 1-15.

Weinberger, Morris, Eugene Z. Oddone, and William G. Henderson. 1996. "Does Increased Access To Primary Care Reduce Hospital Readmissions?" *New England Journal of Medicine* 334 (22): 1441-1447. doi:10.1056/nejm199605303342206.

Weingart, Saul N., Odelya Pagovich, Daniel Z. Sands, Joseph M. Li, Mark D. Aronson, Roger B. Davis, David W. Bates, and Russell S. Phillips. 2005. "What Can Hospitalized Patients Tell Us About Adverse Events? Learning From Patient-Reported Incidents." *Journal of General Internal Medicine* 20 (9): 830-836. doi:10.1111/j.1525-1497.2005.0180.x.

Weissman, Joel S., Eric C. Schneider, Saul N. Weingart, Arnold M. Epstein, JoAnn David-Kasdan, Sandra Feibelmann, Catherine L. Annas, Nancy Ridley, Leslie Kirle, and Constantine Gatsonis. 2008. "Comparing Patient-Reported Hospital Adverse Events With Medical

Record Review: Do Patients Know Something That Hospitals Do Not?" *Annals of Internal Medicine* 149 (2): 100. doi:10.7326/0003-4819-149-2-200807150-00006.

Whittaker, William, Laura Anselmi, Søren Rud Kristensen, Yiu-Shing Lau, Simon Bailey, Peter Bower, and Katherine Checkland et al. 2016. "Associations Between Extending Access To Primary Care And Emergency Department Visits: A Difference-In-Differences Analysis." *PLOS Medicine* 13 (9): e1002113. doi:10.1371/journal.pmed.1002113.

Wigder, Herbert N., Catherine Johnson, Manoj R. Shah, Richard Fantus, Judith Brasic, Kathleen Tanouye, Joan Morris, and Barri Blankenhorn. 2003. "Length Of Stay Predicts Patient And Family Satisfaction With Trauma Center Services." *The American Journal of Emergency Medicine* 21 (7): 606-607. doi:10.1016/j.ajem.2003.08.019.

Wijers, Dorien, Luuk Wieske, Mervyn D. I. Vergouwen, Edo Richard, Jan Stam, and Ellen M. A. Smets. 2010. "Patient Satisfaction In Neurological Second Opinions And Tertiary Referrals." *JournaloOf Neurology* 257 (11): 1869-1874. doi:10.1007/s00415-010-5625-1.

Wilde, Bodil, Gerry Larsson, Mayethel Larsson, and Bengt Starrin. 1994. "Quality Of Care." *Scandinavian Journal of Caring Sciences* 8 (1): 39-48. doi:10.1111/j.1471-6712.1994.tb00223.x.

Wong, Edwin S., Matthew L. Maciejewski, Paul L. Hebert, Ashok Reddy, and Chuan-Fen Liu. 2019. "Predicting Primary Care Use Among Patients In A Large Integrated Health System." *Medical Care* 57 (8): 608-614. doi:10.1097/mlr.0000000000001155.

Wong, Wing S., and Richard Fielding. 2008. "The Association Between Patient Satisfaction And Quality Of Life In Chinese Lung And Liver Cancer Patients." *Medical Care* 46 (3): 293-302. doi:10.1097/mlr.0b013e31815b9785.

Wyshak, Grace, and Arthur Barsky. 1995. "Satisfaction With And Effectiveness Of Medical Care In Relation To Anxiety And Depression." *General Hospital Psychiatry* 17 (2): 108-114. doi:10.1016/0163-8343(94)00097-w.

Xiang Xiao, Wendy Yi Xu, and Randi E. Foraker. 2017. "Is higher patient satisfaction associated with better stroke outcomes?" *The American Journal of Managed Care 23* (10): e316–e322.

Xiao, Hong, and Janet P. Barber. 2008. "The Effect Of Perceived Health Status On Patient Satisfaction." *Value in Health* 11 (4): 719-725. doi:10.1111/j.1524-4733.2007.00294.x.

Xin, Haichang. 2019. "Patient Dissatisfaction With Primary Care And Nonurgent Emergency Department Use." *Journal of Ambulatory Care Management* 42 (4): 284-294. doi:10.1097/jac.0000000000000301.

Yadlapati, Rena, Andrew Gawron, and Rajesh N. Keswani. 2014. "Patient Satisfaction Does Not Correlate With Established Colonoscopy Quality Metrics." *American Journal of Gastroenterology* 109 (7): 1089-1091. doi:10.1038/ajg.2014.115.

Zendjidjian, Xavier, Karine Baumstarck, Pascal Auquier, Anderson Loundou, Christophe Lancon, and Laurent Boyer. 2014. "Satisfaction Of Hospitalized Psychiatry Patients: Why Should Clinicians Care?" *Patient Preference and Adherence*, 575-583. doi:10.2147/ppa.s62278.

Zolnierek, Kelly B. H., and M. Robin DiMatteo. 2009. "Physician Communication And Patient Adherence To Treatment." *Medical Care* 47 (8): 826-834. doi:10.1097/mlr.0b013e31819a5acc.

In: Patient Satisfaction
Editor: Dielle Morneau
ISBN: 978-1-53618-613-0
© 2020 Nova Science Publishers, Inc.

Chapter 2

SATISFACTION WITHIN CHILD AND ADOLESCENT MENTAL HEALTH SERVICE FROM MULTIPLE PERSPECTIVES

Marina Gouhaut[1], Carole Kapp[2], Hélène Beutler[1], Kerstin Jessica von Plessen[2] and Sébastien Urben[2,]**

[1]Child and Adolescent Psychiatry, Hospital of Neuchâtel,
Neuchâtel, Switzerland
[2]Division of Child and Adolescent Psychiatry,
University Hospital of Lausanne, Lausanne, Switzerland

ABSTRACT

Within the context of Child and Adolescent Mental Health Service (CAMHS), patient's and families' satisfaction is of great importance in psychotherapeutic treatment because it is closely linked to positive clinical improvements as well as to subsequent requests for help. Furthermore, the integration of multiple perspectives (e.g., children/adolescents, parents, clinicians) is of crucial importance. Therefore, in this chapter we will, first, describe the instruments used to

---

* Corresponding Author's E-mail: Sebastien.Urben@chuv.ch.

assess satisfaction. Afterwards, we will focus on the presentation of the various factors related to satisfaction in the field of child and adolescent psychiatry. In particular, we will focus on the determinants such as the intra-individual characteristics, the inter-personal dimensions, treatment outcomes, the organization of care/services and the expectations. More specifically, we will describe these factors from different perspectives (i.e., children/adolescents, parents, clinicians) and in different types of treatment (i.e., out- and inpatient). The last part of the chapter will be devoted to identifying the limits in identifying satisfaction determinants and proposing avenues for future researches. The chapter is enriched by clinical examples to illustrate the described theoretical aspects.

Keywords: child and adolescent mental health service, satisfaction, multiple informants, determinants

INTRODUCTION

"I can't get no satisfaction" taken from the famous song of the Rolling Stones released in 1965, which made and continues to make generations of individuals dance, tells us the story from one side of a society of opulence and euphoria in the 60s and another left behind who did not feel at home in the society. Although, it introduced the concept of frustration and hence of dissatisfaction, which did not tarnish according to the time, it also allowed thinking about elements satisfying people.

Looking at the Latin etymology of the word satisfaction satis- adverb which means "sufficient"/"which is suitable, good" and substantive faction corresponding to the verb "facere" which means "to do," therefore satisfaction refers to "to do the right thing." However, how do we know if, what is done, is right and will bring satisfaction? This question is of highest importance in today's society, which is based on the wish to be always more efficient and to respond in an increasingly personalized way to consumer's demands. The notion of satisfaction get increased interests in the health sector striving to offer personalized medicine by adapting the care to the rhythm of the patient and their relatives.

The World Health Organization (WHO) estimated that one in five children and adolescents has a mental disorder and that about half of mental disorders begin before the age of 14 (WHO 2019). This should make children and adolescents mental health a public health priority. Therefore, we have to be able not only to prevent, but also to optimize the care of children and adolescents suffering from psychopathological difficulties. In particular, child and adolescent psychiatry regroups mainly two types of care: the outpatient treatment (e.g., ambulatory treatment, community treatment) and the inpatient treatment (i.e., hospital).

The care of the outpatient child and adolescent psychiatry consultation consists of welcoming not only children and adolescents suffering from psychological difficulties, but also their parents. The care begins with an anamnesis of the patients and their family and a detailed examination of the mental health of the child or the adolescent in a specific family context. Psychological investigations in the form of tests are often carried out. According to the established diagnosis, a treatment plan is proposed, and organized with the patients and their families. Therapists (e.g., psychiatrists and/or psychologists) provide supportive treatment, guidance, therapeutic consultations, psychotherapy, family follow-up or group therapy.

The inpatient treatment consists of taking care of patients in crisis or emergency situations for whom the care provided in an ambulatory setting is not sufficient (i.e., outpatient treatment). The hospital setting provides a safe environment adapted to the individual needs of each patient. The objectives are defined in collaboration with the children and adolescents, as well as the parents and professionals who support them. A multidisciplinary team consisting usually of child psychiatrists, psychologists, nurses, teacher, educators and sometimes a hospital pediatric team supervise the patient during hospitalization. The patient may benefit from individual, family and network interviews, workshops and mediated therapeutic activities as well as academic support.

Herein, we focus on the satisfaction of the users in child and adolescent mental health services (CAMHS) because it is linked, among others, to positive clinical improvements as well as their subsequent uses of service (Fitzpatrick 1993). However, the factors determining satisfaction are not yet well understood. In addition, we will focus on the integration of multiple perspectives (i.e., children/adolescents, parents and clinicians), as it is crucial in this context of care. Indeed, this triad has to resonate in unison as the three chords of the song of the Rolling stones cited at the beginning of this chapter.

Moreover, according to the WHO "mental health strategies and intervention for treatment, prevention and promotion need to be based on scientific evidence and/or best practice, taking cultural consideration into account" (WHO 2013). In this line, the concept of evidence-based practice is crucial. Evidence-based practice allow to take the best clinical decision based on the up-to-date available clinical evidence, the clinician's expertise and the patients' specificities (Sackett et al. 1996).

First, we will review the different instruments allowing assessing satisfaction within CAMHS. Then, we will describe the factors influencing the satisfaction within CAMHS, taking into account the various perspectives (i.e., patients, parents, clinicians) and the type of treatment (i.e., out- and inpatient). Moreover, the chapter is enriched by clinical examples illustrating the described theoretical aspects.

INSTRUMENTS OF MEASURES

Clinical Example

Nina, a 16-year-old girl followed for anxiety symptomatology for 6 months shows signs of depression: persistent fatigue, loss of motivation, increased irritability. The therapist shared her own thoughts with Nina in favor of a diagnosis of depression. Nina was satisfied with the care, so far, but suddenly felt judged and devalued in that a psychiatric diagnosis was made without trying to take into account the recent elements that have led to this state for a week (e.g., her boyfriend left her, she failed an important school exam).

This case highlighted the complexity and the importance of attentive listening and the necessity of an overall vision of the patient and empathy in the interaction. Thinking of satisfaction referred to understand the patient as a whole (in terms of her/his person, her/his health, her/his family, her/his relatives, her/his education, her/his hobbies, etc.) to be able to have the most accurate representation of her/him. Moreover, this example illustrates that satisfaction was not a static factor in a relationship, but refers to a dynamic process that should be carefully taken into account throughout the therapeutical process.

The use of valid tools or instruments with known psychometrics properties allows comparing the level of satisfaction across studies and discuss their results built on the same basis. Therefore, we will describe the main instruments that enable to measure satisfaction in out- and inpatient (see Table 1 below).

In general, it is important to distinguish between quantitative and qualitative surveys. Within quantitative surveys, questionnaires have been developed that allow to measure satisfaction either as a global satisfaction or focusing on some specific aspects. In qualitative surveys, however, specific open-ended questions are developed for the purpose of the particular study. This allows to go in more details in the understanding of satisfaction regarding a specific treatment received within CAMHS.

One of the most used questionnaire in studies of satisfaction in child and adolescent mental health in inpatient and outpatient care was the Client Satisfaction Questionnaire (CSQ-8; Larsen et al. 1979). The CSQ-8 included eight items that were chosen based on assessments by mental health professionals of a number of items that could be related to client satisfaction and by a subsequent factor analysis. The CSQ-8 is unidimensional, which allowed a uniform estimate of general satisfaction with the services (Kapp et al. 2014). It is available in more than 30 languages.

Table 1. Description of the quantitative instruments

Questionnaire :	#Items; scale(s):	Versions for :
Consumer Satisfaction Questionnaire (CSQ-8) (Larsen et al. 1979)	8 items; - Global satisfaction	Child/Adolescent Parent
Experience of service questionnaire ESQ (Brown et al. 2014)	15 items; - Facilities - Staff - How well the patient was treated - Confidence in staff - Overall satisfaction with the service	Child/Adolescent Parent
Multidimensional Adolescent Satisfaction Scale (MASS) (Mathiesen, Cash, and Hudson 2002)	21 items; - Counselor qualities - Meeting needs - Effectiveness - Counselor conflict	Child/Adolescent
The CAMHS Satisfaction Scale outpatient (CAMHSSS) (Ayton et al. 2007)	Versions with 20 or 39 items; - Overall satisfaction - Professionals' skills and behaviour - Information - Accessibility of services - Effectiveness of treatment - Relatives' involvement - Types of intervention offered	Child/Adolescent Parent Therapist

Questionnaire :	#Items; scale(s):	Versions for :
Hospital's Perception of Care (POC) survey (Madan et al. 2016)	20 items; - Interpersonal aspects of care - Continuity/coordination of care - Communication/Information received from treatment providers - Global evaluation of care	Child/Adolescent Parent

Another tool assessing the general experience of patients and their parents was the service experience questionnaire (ESQ; Brown et al. 2014) developed by the Health Improvement Commission of the time (now the Health Care Commission) to measure satisfaction with services in mental health services for children and adolescents. The ESQ was originally used as an anonymous measure for spot audits of service delivery, but the Child Outcomes Research Consortium advises that it should be used regularly in combination with other basic measures so that a family's experiences with the service can be understood alongside the reduction of the child's symptoms (Brown et al. 2014). The ESQ consisted of 12 elements and three sections of free text examining what the respondent liked about the service, what he felt he needed to improve and any other comments.

The Multidimensional Adolescent Satisfaction Scale (MASS), the CAMHS Satisfaction Scale outpatient (CAMHSSS-20 and CAMHSSS-39) or the CAMHS Satisfaction Scale inpatient (CAMHSSS-Uni) have been adapted from the Verona Service Satisfaction Scale (Ruggeri et al. 1996). There exist four versions, a short version with 20 items; a long version with 39 items more adapted for research or service developments (Ayton et al. 2007) and version for inpatient (CAMHSSS-Uni, also with 20 or 39 items). Another instrument for satisfaction specifically dedicated to inpatient was the hospital's Perception of Care (POC) survey.

However, the above described instruments focus on a general evaluation and often lack finesse and details which was a limitation of the quantitive studies. By contrats, qualitative surveys could bring us more subtleties and subjectivity (Biering and Jensen 2017). They were based on semi-structured interviews, which necessitate then thematic analysis (Coyne and al. 2015). Therefore, qualitative surveys might be adapted to the specific need and context of studies. However, such results were less easily comparable.

SATISFACTION FACTORS

"But what are these "throw-ins," these elusive, "off the record." extras?"- Irvin Yalom (1980)

According to the principle of John Stuart Mill (Mill 1863), an action is considered "good" when it increases happiness or when it reduces the overall suffering of (wo)men. To evaluate morally an action, we have to take into account not only the intention, but also the consequences. Thus, the means employed and the result achieved should be in coherence.

Next, we reviewed the studies examining the determinants of satisfaction (see Table 2 below). The studies were retrieved from Pubmed with keywords such as "satisfaction", "child and adolescent psychiatry", "child and mental health service," "outpatient" and "inpatient." Moreover, the bibliography of each selected studies has been screened to select other important studies (i.e., backward search strategy) that described satisfaction determinants within CAMHS and thus warranted inclusion in the selection of this literature review.

Thirty-one studies have been conducted to examine the determinants of satisfaction. In particular, in outpatient context, we observed, that, out of 18 in total, 12 studies integrated the patient's point of view (n = 3), 14 studies assessed the parents' point of view (n = 3250) and four studies examined the therapists' point of view (n = 148). Three studies were merely qualitative (Coyne et al. 2015, Widmark et al. 2013, Wisdom et al. 2011), whereas the others adopted a quantitative methodology. The number of participants varied between five and 2164. Six of these studies focused on a specific psychopathology (e.g., disruptive behaviors problems, anxiety or depression, substance abuse, eating disorders and antisocial behaviors).

In the studies carried out in inpatient setting, out of eight studies in total, we observed that six integrated the point of view of the child/adolescents (n = 607), seven studies assessed the parents' point of view (n = 319) and no study examined the clinician's point of view. Two studies were only qualitative (Katzenschlager and al. 2018, Biering and al.

2011), the other studies adopted a quantitative methodology or a mix one. Only one of these studies focused on a specific pathology, schizophrenia spectrum disorders. The number of participants varied between 14 and 211.

In the mix studies (including out- and inpatient surveys), out of five studies in total, we observed that three integrated the patient's point of view (n = 5894), three studies assessed the parents' point of view (n = 59) and no study examined the therapists' point of view. One study (Persson, Hagquist, and Michelson 2017) included qualitative survey while the others studies were quantitative or mix. The number of pariticipants varied between 48 and 4345.

According to a previous review of literature (Biering 2010) aiming at synthesizing the perception of the quality of psychiatric care for children and adolescents, three main components influenced satisfaction: (a) the relationship with professionals (i.e., acceptance/understanding, empathy/friendliness, listening/attending skills and non-judgmental approach for therapist), (b) the environment/organization of CAMHS (i.e., accessibility, comfort/cleanliness of the service) and (c) the treatment outcomes (i.e., positives changes in thoughts, feelings and behaviors).

The present review of literature shed some light on this previous literature review. The more recent studies, led us to think that the Biering's assumptions remained partially valid. However, we had to go a step further by specifying the determinants and adding new components. Indeed, from our literature review, the determinants of satisfaction might be grouped into (a) the intra-individual characteristics of the patient or the parents (e.g., age, gender, overall functioning, psychopathologies); (b) the inter-individual variables such as the therapist's relationship with the patient and family (e.g., treatment, information and communication); (c) the environment/organization of the service (e.g., environment, access); (d) the treatment outcomes and (e) the expectations about future, such as prognosis (Garland, Haine, and Boxmeyer 2007, Viefhaus et al. 2019) or about the way the treatment should be done (e.g., personalization of care) (Kapp et al. 2017). Below, we will specify each determinant.

Table 2. Determinants of satisfaction in function of the type of CAMHS treatment

Type of treatment	Study	N	Factors influencing satisfaction
Outpatient	Viefhaus et al. (2020)	Patient: 795	- Treatment variables (i.e., status at treatment end, symptom improvement) - Type of diagnoses - Evolution of mental health problems pre- and post-assessment - Parent's qualities of relationships with peers - Educational level of mother - Parent's cooperation - Therapist training
	Man and Kangas (2019)	Parent: 41	- Role of parent - Support for family - Distrust of caregiver
	Défayes et al. (2019)	Patient: 69	- Children's right
	Viefhaus et al. (2019)	Patient: 956	- Evolution of mental health problems pre- and post-assessment - Patient rating of the evolution of their difficulties - Number of children in the patient's family - Qualities of upbringing - Parent's cooperation - Patient's cooperation - The number of parent/family focus intervention - Sociotherapeutic interventions - Prognosis for the overall situation - Number of treatment sessions - Treatment came to a regular end

Table 2. (Continued)

Type of treatment	Study	N	Factors influencing satisfaction
	Kapp et al. (2017)	Parents: 770 Patient: 663	- Approach to treatment (i.e., reassurance at the first appointment - patient and parent -, agreement for the first appointment - patient) - Satisfaction with the frequency of sessions - Time to ask questions
	Accurso and Garland (2015)	Patient: 209 Therapist: 85	- Therapist training - Racial/ethnic of therapist - Therapeutic alliance
	Coyne et al. (2015)	Patient: 15 Parent: 32	- Information - Relationship between families and professionals - Parenting courses - Collaboration - Clinician continuity
	Widmark et al. (2013)	Patient: 7 Parent: 5	- Quality of contact (i.e., availability, information, empathy, openness, commitment, professionals' skills, parents' efforts) - Strength of collaboration (i.e., coordination among the professionals, communication links, joint meetings)
	Wisdom et al. (2011)	Patient: 28 Parent: 30 Staff: 24	- Cost and medical insurance - Wait time - Motivation - Denial - Educating families - Support for patient and family

Type of treatment	Study	N	Factors influencing satisfaction
			- Stigma - Lack of awareness about the youth's substance abuse - Acknowledge patient's problems - Family's experience - Awareness and understanding of the treatment process and options
	Zaitsoff and Taylor (2009)	Patient: 54 only girls	- Characteristics of the parent-adolescent relationship - Severity eating disorder
	Bjorngaard et al. (2008)	Parent: 2164	- Patient's age - Clinician abilities (i.e., care, understanding, trust, knowledge) - Information provide - Treatment outcome
	Garland, Haine, and Boxmeyer (2007)	Patient: 143 Families: 223	- Patient functional impairment - Patient race/ethnicity - Treatment expectations - Caregiver strain - Therapist's years of experience - Number of treatment sessions
	Barber, Tischler, and Healy (2006)	Patient: 45 Parent: 73	- Treatment engagement - Therapist engagement - Quality of life
	Garcia and Weisz (2002)	Families: 344	- Therapeutic relationship - Money issues

Table 2. (Continued)

Type of treatment	Study	N	Factors influencing satisfaction
	Garland et al. (2000)	Patient: 180	- Adolescent's attitudes - Severity of mental health problems - Adolescent's choice/motivation - Expectation about services
	Kazdin and Wassell (2000)	Patient and their family: 157	- Parent psychopathology - Quality of life
	Kazdin, Holland, and Crowley (1997)	242 children and families	- Coming to treatment - Relationship between parent and therapist - Socioeconomic situation - Family circumstances - Parent history - Child history
	Urben et al. (2015)	Patient: 20 Foster carers: 19 Professional caregiver: 39	- Relationship with patient - Observation every day - Clinical outcome : emotional symptoms - Patients stay in their community - Flexibility
Inpatient	Galitzer et al. (2020)	Patient: 211	- Satisfaction is similar with non-psychotic disorder - Medication - Need longer admissions - More extended clinical input
	Katzenschlager et al. (2018)	Patient: 50	- Parental involvement - Information

Type of treatment	Study	N	Factors influencing satisfaction
	Madan et al. (2016)	Patient: 129 Parent: 101	- Patient (i.e., secure place, tough love, peer solidarity, self-expression, and person not patient) - Child behaviors as assessed by parents
	Biering and Jensen (2011)	Patient: 14	- Secure place - Keep connection with family, friends and school - Sports and physical activities - Tough love and discipline - Peer solidarity - Express their feelings - Treated as person not as a patient - Family relations
	Tas, Guvenir, and Cevrim (2010)	Patient: 46	- Information about treatment and the physical conditions of the service - Information about psychological problems - The expected treatment outcome and expected side effects - Staff - The treatment environment - Food, meaning of meal
	Blader (2007)	Parent: 107	- Child behavior trouble - Perception of inpatient experience
	Kaplan et al. (2001)	Patient: 157 Parent/guardian: 111	- Staff behavior - Improvement of the problem

Table 2. (Continued)

Type of treatment	Study	N	Factors influencing satisfaction
	Bradley and Clark (1993)	56 children and their family	- Including parent - Staff's lack of attention to their home-based problems - Communication - Opportunities for reviewing the progress of treatment - Voicing concerns
Mix (out- and inpatient)	Lindstedt, Kjellin, and Gustafsson (2017)	Patient: 4345	- Individual therapy - Family therapy - Most important goal: "to learn to eat normally" - Working with rigid thoughts and underlying psychosocial factor - Therapist's ability to help them and to understand their problems - Patient's participation - Treatment interventions focusing on body image, self-perception and emotion regulation
	Persson, Hagquist, and Michelson (2017)	Patient: Qualitative: 7 Quantitative: 106	- Accessible services - Communication openly - Participation session activities - Relationship with the therapist - Environment - Listens and validates their point of view - Overt emphasis on balancing the views of parents - External pressure - Adolescent preferred creative ways of conveying their feelings and problems - Choice of appointment times

Type of treatment	Study	N	Factors influencing satisfaction
	Halvorsen and Heyerdahl (2007)	Patient: 48 only girls Mother: 33 Father: 26	- Family therapy - Therapeutic alliance - *"Willpower"*, *"Wish to recover"* and *"Readiness for change"* - Support from the mother - External support for mother - Information and support parents had received - Patient's age at start of treatment for parent
	Stacey et al. (2002)	Parent: 110	- Evolution of mental health problems pre- and post- assessment - Treated with respect, understanding their situation and do new paths for action - Managing, supporting and strengthening parent
	Rey, Plapp, and Simpson (1999)	Patient: 1278	- Time of treatment - Information - Relationship

Intra-Individual Characteristics

Patients reported that satisfaction may decrease when they get older, with relationships becoming more confrontational while entering adolescence (Garland, Haine, and Boxmeyer 2007). Parents reported equally, as the age of their children at the start of treatment might contribute to better satisfaction if children are younger (Viefhaus et al. 2019) and less satisfied if they are older (Bjorngaard et al. 2008). Patient' psychopathology (Viefhaus et al. 2020), as well as parent's psychopathology (Kazdin and Wassell 2000) was of importance to understand satisfaction. In particular, parents whose children had externalizing disorders were often less satisfied (Viefhaus et al. 2020). Additionally, other factors related to satisfaction were the characteristics of the child such as history, educational level, experiences, functioning, socioeconomic situation, stigma and the awareness and understanding of the treatment process and options as well as the adolescent's attitude (Garland et al. 2000, Kazdin, Holland, and Crowley 1997, Kazdin and Wassell 2000, Viefhaus et al. 2020, Wisdom et al. 2011). Within, the inpatient treatment, from parent's point of view, child's functioning and their development during care (Blader 2007, Madan et al. 2016) were an important source of satisfaction. Moreover, a study focusing on a particular type of diagnosis, namely schizophrenia spectrum disorders (Galitzer et al. 2020), observed that the patient may be satisfied with the medication. The child functioning (from the parent's point of view) was a criterion of satisfaction in a study including out- and inpatient sample (Stacey et al. 2002). A study observed that the *"Willpower,"* *"Wish to recover"* and *"Readiness for change"* (Halvorsen and Heyerdahl 2007) as well as patient's participation (Lindstedt, Kjellin, and Gustafsson 2017) were important determinants of satisfaction.

Inter-Individual Variables

From patients' perspective, the quality of the relationship with the therapist and the respect of the child's right (Défayes et al. 2019, Persson, Hagquist, and Michelson 2017, Shirk and Karver 2003) referred to important factors for satisfaction. Noticed that patients reported that the therapeutic alliance were stable over time but therapist reported variability and difference in function of the patients (Accurso and Garland 2015). Likewise, the continuity of care (i.e., same therapist) as well as the availability of the therapist was important to understand satisfaction (Coyne et al. 2015). In this line, patients were sensitive to the experience of the therapist (Garland, Haine, and Boxmeyer 2007) or therapist training (Accurso and Garland 2015, Viefhaus et al. 2020). From the parent's point of view, satisfaction predictors referred to the quality of the first contact (Kapp et al. 2017), cooperation with the therapist (Accurso and Garland 2015, Coyne et al. 2015, Viefhaus et al. 2019, 2020), support of their parenthood (Coyne et al. 2015, Man and Kangas 2019, Wisdom et al. 2011) as well as by the therapist's skills and professional experience (Accurso and Garland 2015, Bjorngaard et al. 2008, Garland, Haine, and Boxmeyer 2007). Moreover, the therapeutic relationship between them and the therapist (Accurso and Garland 2015, Coyne et al. 2015, Garcia and Weisz 2002, Kazdin, Holland, and Crowley 1997, Widmark et al. 2013) as well as the information and communication (Coyne et al. 2015, Garcia and Weisz 2002, Widmark et al. 2013, Wisdom et al. 2011) were important determinants of satisfaction.

Within inpatient treatment, information and communication about the treatment and the pathology were important determinant of satisfaction, reported by patients and their parents, (Bradley and Clark 1993, Katzenschlager et al. 2018, Tas, Guvenir, and Cevrim 2010). A recent study reported that the most satisfied parents were those who were involved in the therapeutic process proposed to their child (Katzenschlager et al. 2018). Finally, the attention and staff behavior towards parents were reported in three of five studies (Bradley and Clark 1993, Kaplan et al.

2001, Tas, Guvenir, and Cevrim 2010) as important determinants of satisfaction.

Likewise, the relationship with the therapist with the opportunity to communicate openly was observed as an important factor of satisfaction in two studies including out- and inpatient samples (Halvorsen and Heyerdahl 2007, Persson, Hagquist, and Michelson 2017). In particular, the relationship between parents and the therapist (Rey, Plapp, and Simpson 1999) and between patient and therapist (Halvorsen and Heyerdahl 2007) as well as information and support (Halvorsen and Heyerdahl 2007, Rey, Plapp, and Simpson 1999, Stacey et al. 2002) referred to important determinants of satisfaction. Moreover, the therapist's ability to help them and to understand their problems was crucial to enhance satisfaction (Lindstedt, Kjellin, and Gustafsson 2017).

Treatment Outcomes

Lower symptoms at the end of the treatment were related to higher satisfaction (Garland, Haine, and Boxmeyer 2007, Stacey et al. 2002, Viefhaus et al. 2019). Likewise, treatment outcomes were also an important factor of satisfaction for parents (Bjorngaard et al. 2008, Garland, Haine, and Boxmeyer 2007, Kazdin, Holland, and Crowley 1997, Viefhaus et al. 2019, 2020).

Environment/Organization of the Service

Longer waiting times before the first appointment were a source of dissatisfaction, especially among the youngest children (Biering and Jensen 2011). Moreover, the higher the numbers of sessions, the higher the satisfaction, however, this is coupled with the fact that the treatment come to a regular end (Viefhaus et al. 2019) and thus it is not possible to disentangle the reason and the consequence in this case. Financial issues (e.g., cost and medical insurance difficulties) might reduce satisfaction (Garcia and Weisz 2002, Wisdom et al. 2011).

Inpatient surveys revealed that the daily routine (rituals of getting up and going to bed and the schedules punctuating the day) were an important source of satisfaction (Tas, Guvenir, and Cevrim 2010). Moreover, voicing concerns might impair satisfaction (Bradley and Clark 1993).

Finally, in a mix survey (including out- and inpatient), accessibility and environment has been observed to be an important factor of satisfaction (Persson, Hagquist, and Michelson 2017). Moreover, the treatment interventions focusing on body image, self-perception and emotion regulation might help to enhance satisfaction (Lindstedt, Kjellin, and Gustafsson 2017).

Expectations

Representation of the future seems to be an important factor to understand satisfaction. Indeed, a better prognosis increased satisfaction, which was important for parents and patients (Viefhaus et al. 2019). As well, patients expectation about services (e.g., type of site where the treatment is given) (Garland et al. 2000) was a determinant of satisfaction. Enhanced satisfaction was observed in patients who had more time to ask questions, who were satisfied with the frequency of the appointment (Kapp et al. 2017) and who had the choice of appointment times (Persson, Hagquist, and Michelson 2017). In other words, the more personalized the treatment were the more satisfied the patient were. In this line, the flexibility of treatment (Urben et al. 2015) or the creative ways of conveying their feelings and problems (Persson, Hagquist, and Michelson 2017) led to higher satisfaction.

Inpatient surveys revealed that parents wanted to be respected, listened, and received the appropriate help (Vusio et al. 2019). Likewise, patients wanted to be considered as a person and not as a patient and patients expected to be respected, to be listen to, to be able to express himself or herself and to feel safe (Biering and Jensen 2011, Madan et al.

2016). Moreover, patients wished to maintain a link with their outside world as well as with their family, peers, school and activities and that during the care (Biering and Jensen 2011) which led to higher satisfaction.

Mix surveys (including out- and inpatient) revealed that the participation of the patient in the treatment led to higher satisfaction when evaluating the significance of the treatment (Lindstedt, Kjellin, and Gustafsson 2017, Persson, Hagquist, and Michelson 2017).

MULTIPLE PERSPECTIVES

Clinical Example

Peter, an adolescent of 17 years of age attending CAMHS for lowered thymia and sleep disturbances in emergency on request of his parents. He was the only child of the parental couple. His mother did not work because of a leg disability, she also had psychiatric treatment due to depression. His father was an engineer. There was no contact with maternal or paternal grandparents.

Parents during their sessions, drew the picture of an inert adolescent under the consumption of alcohol and cannabis. Parents were very worried and asked for medication for their son (their only request) and insisted for drug treatment.

On the adolescent side, we observed a young man in bond who struggles to express what he felt and who described a complex family climate and his parents as alcoholics. The psychiatric assessment did not give any indication for drug treatment but for treatment by intensive supportive therapy.

The parents did not agree with the care and the diagnostic hypothesis. The parents said that their son wanted treatment, which was not the case during individual sessions with the patient. Parents were not satisfied with the care. The demands became so intrusive that Paul said he felt a conflict of loyalty between the indications of the therapist and his parents' insistence on medication. He could not fully invest his therapeutic space even if he remained satisfied with the current care. A collaborative communication with the parents allowed them to explain that for them in their personal care, medication was the most helpful, and therefore wanted the same care for their son. From that point on, the collaboration between the therapist and the family has been enhanced and, thus, the process of care developed more efficiently.

This case makes us particularly attentive to the attitude of parents who showed insistence on the implementation of treatment for their son. In child psychiatry, it is common for parents to wish a medication thinking that it could be an optimal treatment for the difficulties because they often feel helpless and want their children to be relieved immediately. Parents had to be considered in their entirety (their life history, their health, their profession, their vision of their child) and to understand their apprehension of child's psychopathology. Additionally, this case illustrated how important the various perspectives (i.e., youths, parents and therapist) should be taken into account in order to enhance satisfaction.

More generally, studies reported patients are generally less satisfied than their parents (Katzenschlager et al. 2018, Madan et al. 2016) or fostercarer (Urben et al. 2015), and therapists are generally less satisfied than parents (Viefhaus et al. 2020) or fostercarer (Urben et al. 2015).

PROSPECTS FOR USE/DISCUSSION

We could see through this chapter that it was a challenge to draw firm conclusions concerning the determinants of satisfaction. Indeed, gray areas were still to be explored. Studies including multifocal views were scarce, but seemed promising to enhance the understanding of satisfaction within CAMHS. The therapists' point of view remained in majority not taken into account and thus unexamined. To the best of our knowledge, no factors were examined to understand their satisfaction or dissatisfaction with the therapy they are involved in. Little evidence exists on what parents perceive as satisfaction factors in their children's perception.

Some elements seemed to have their importance depending on the pathology, such as family therapy as a factor of satisfaction in the management of eating disorders (Halvorsen and Heyerdahl 2007, Lindstedt, Kjellin, and Gustafsson 2017), collaboration between professionals in the management of depression or anxiety (Widmark et al. 2013) or motivation among young people with substance use (Wisdom et al. 2011). Thus, further studies are warranted to affine these preliminary findings.

The therapeutic relationship (or alliance) played an important role in satisfaction (Biering 2010, Shirk and Karver 2003). Likewise, expectations about the therapist (Karver et al. 2006), as well as the desire of parents and patients to be able to be treated as a person, to be listened to and respected (Vusio et al. 2019) seemed to emerge as crucial factors. Nevertheless, we did not know what allowed the patient to feel welcomed and listened to and, how may the therapist respond to these important expectations. This also should be examined in future studies. Moreover, how the patients understood the information transmitted by the therapist, which also played a crucial role (e.g., Reardon et al. 2017), should be further studied. Another element, which need further examination, was the specification of communication, verbally but also body language, within the many interactions in a care.

Regarding the settings (out- and inpatient), there seemed that both type of treatment lead to satisfaction and that the determinants did not seems to be very different for each treatment. Satisfaction seemed to emerge from the collaboration between the patient and the parents (i.e., the family as a whole entity), as well as the professional network (which should be included in future researches). Satisfaction is therefore not for one but for several people, each with different needs and expectations, which introduces the complexity of developing individualized care making sense for everyone. Moreover, satisfaction is dynamic and can evolve during the treatment process (Accurso and Garland 2015).

CONCLUSION

Throughout this chapter, we realized the challenges to identify the general determinants of satisfaction, as well as the complexity of the different points of view that should be in coherence to lead to satisfactory treatment. One of the factors that came up most often is the relationship with the therapist. It would therefore be important to assess this relationship from a multifocal point of view including the vision of the patient, parents and therapists. One of the important points in this relationship is the identification of the patient's feelings (e.g., perception, understanding and expression). If the patient might feel to be misunderstood, it would then be necessary to specify and to understand what she / he express. It is not uncommon that if you take a metaphor or quote as an example, people could understand different aspects of it, which is why it is important to compare its aspects so that everyone can understand the other perspective. The understanding of words, the transmission of information are important elements, but let's not forget that the attitude of the body is also important . Thus, the number of variables that are taken into account in the perception of satisfaction accounts for the complexity of being able to generalize this feeling. Especially, as the needs differ from one person to another. Therefore, further studies might identify more specific or presonalized determinants of satisfaction.

However, some determinants, that should be further specified, seem to emerge from our literature review: (a) the intra-individual characteristics; (b) the inter-individual variables; (c) the environment / organization of the service (e.g., environment, access); (d) the treatment outcomes and (e) the expectations. Nevertheless, it is therefore important to be able to continue researches in this area in order to provide the most individualized care possible in order to meet the closest needs of our patients and their families.

> "Whatever the progress of human knowledge, there will always be room for ignorance and therefore for chance and probability." (Borel 1914)

REFERENCES

Accurso, E. C., and A. F. Garland. 2015. "Child, Caregiver, and Therapist Perspectives on Therapeutic Alliance in Usual Care Child Psychotherapy." *Psychological Assessment* 27 (1):347-352. doi: 10.1037/pas0000031.

Ayton, A. K., M. P. Mooney, K. Sillifant, J. Powls, and H. Rasool. 2007. "The development of the child and adolescent versions of the Verona Service Satisfaction Scale (CAMHSSS)." *Social psychiatry and psychiatric epidemiology* 42:892-901.

Barber, A. J., V. A. Tischler, and E. Healy. 2006. "Consumer Satisfaction and Child Behaviour Problems in Child and Adolescent Mental Health Services." *Journal of Child Health Care: For Professionals Working with Children in the Hospital and Community* 10:9-21. doi: 10.1177/1367493506060200.

Biering, P. 2010. "Child and adolescent experience of and satisfaction with psychiatric care: a critical review of the research literature." *Journal of Psychiatric and Mental Health Nursing* 17 (1):65-72. doi: 10.1111/j.1365-2850.2009.01505.x.

Biering, P., and V. H. Jensen. 2011. "The Concept of Patient Satisfaction in Adolescent Psychiatric Care: A Qualitative Study." *Journal of Child and Adolescent Psychiatric Nursing: Official Publication of the Association of Child and Adolescent Psychiatric Nurses* 24:3-10. doi: 10.1111/j.1744-6171.2010.00261.x.

Biering, P., and V. H. Jensen. 2017. "The concept of patient satisfaction in adolescent psychiatric care: A qualitative study." *Journal of Child and Adolescent Psychiatric Nursing* 30 (4):162-169. doi: 10.1111/jcap.12189.

Bjorngaard, J. H., H. W. Andersson, S. O. Ose, and K. Hanssen-Bauer. 2008. "User satisfaction with child and adolescent mental health services - Impact of the service unit level." *Social Psychiatry and Psychiatric Epidemiology* 43 (8):635-641. doi: 10.1007/s00127-008-0347-8.

Blader, J. C. 2007. "Longitudinal assessment of parental satisfaction with children's psychiatric hospitalization." *Administration and Policy in Mental Health and Mental Health Services Research* 34 (2):108-115. doi: 10.1007/s10488-006-0085-8.

Borel, E. 1914. *Le Hasard*. Paris: Nouvelle collection scientifique. [*Chance*]

Bradley, E. J., and B. S. Clark. 1993. "Patients Characteristics and Consumer Satisfaction on an Inpatient Child Psychiatric Unit." *Canadian Journal of Psychiatry-Revue Canadienne De Psychiatrie* 38 (3):175-180. doi: 10.1177/070674379303800304.

Brown, A., T. Ford, J. Deighton, and W. Wolpert. 2014. "Satisfaction in Child and Adolescent Mental Health Services." *Administration and Policy in Mental Health and Mental Health Services Research* 41:436-446.

Coyne, I., N. McNamara, M. Healy, C. Gower, M. Sarkar, and F. McNicholas. 2015. "Adolescents' and parents' views of Child and Adolescent Mental Health Services (CAMHS) in Ireland." *Journal of Psychiatric and Mental Health Nursing* 22 (8):561-569. doi: 10.1111/jpm.12215.

Défayes, F., S. Habersaat, S. Urben, P. D. Jaffé, and C. Kapp. 2019. "Apport d'une perspective « droits de l'enfant » dans les prises en charge ambulatoires en psychiatrie de l'adolescent." *Enfance* 81:152-165. [Contribution of a "rights of the child" perspective to outpatient treatment in adolescent psychiatry.]

Fitzpatrick, R. 1993. "Scope and measurement of patient satisfaction." In *Measurement of patients' satisfaction with their care*, edited by R. Fitzpatrick and A. Hopkins, 1-17. London: Royal College of Physicians.

Galitzer, H., N. Anagnostopoulou, A. Alba, J. Gaete, D. Dima, and M. Kyriakopoulos. 2020. "Functional outcomes and patient satisfaction following inpatient treatment for childhood-onset schizophrenia spectrum disorders vs non-psychotic disorders in children in the United Kingdom." *Early Intervention in Psychiatry*. doi: 10.1111/eip.12973.

Garcia, J. A., and J. R. Weisz. 2002. "When youth mental health care stops: Therapeutic relationship problems and other reasons for ending youth outpatient treatment." *Journal of Consulting and Clinical Psychology* 70 (2):439-443. doi: 10.1037//0022-006x.70.2.439.

Garland, A. F., G. A. Aarons, M. D. Saltzman, and M. I. Kruse. 2000. "Correlates of Adolescents' Satisfaction with Mental Health Services." *Mental Health Services Research* 2:127-139.

Garland, A. F., R. A. Haine, and C. L. Boxmeyer. 2007. "Determinates of youth and parent satisfaction in usual care psychotherapy." *Evaluation and Program Planning* 30 (1):45-54. doi: 10.1016/j.evalprogplan.2006.10.003.

Halvorsen, I., and S. Heyerdahl. 2007. "Treatment perception in adolescent onset anorexia nervosa: Retrospective views of patients and parents." *International Journal of Eating Disorders* 40 (7):629-639. doi: 10.1002/eat.20428.

Kaplan, S., J. Busner, J. Chibnall, and G. Kang. 2001. "Consumer satisfaction at a child and adolescent state psychiatric hospital." *Psychiatric Services* 52 (2):202-206. doi: 10.1176/appi.ps.52.2.202.

Kapp, C., T. Perlini, S. Baggio, P. Stephan, A. R. Urrego, C. E. Rengade, M. Macias, N. Hainard, and O. Halfon. 2014. "Psychometric properties of the Consumer Satisfaction Questionnaire (CSQ-8) and the Helping Alliance Questionnaire (HAQ)." *Sante Publique* 26 (3):337-344. doi: 10.3917/spub.139.0337.

Kapp, C., T. Perlini, T. Jeanneret, P. Stephan, A. Rojas-Urrego, M. Macias, O. Halfon, L. Holzer, and S. Urben. 2017. "Identifying the determinants of perceived quality in outpatient child and adolescent mental health services from the perspectives of parents and patients." *European Child & Adolescent Psychiatry* 26 (10):1269-1277. doi: 10.1007/s00787-017-0985-z.

Karver, M. S., J. B. Handelsman, S. Fields, and L. Bickman. 2006. "Meta-analysis of therapeutic relationship variables in youth and family therapy: The evidence for different relationship variables in the child and adolescent treatment outcome literature." *Clinical Psychology Review* 26 (1):50-65. doi: 10.1016/j.cpr.2005.09.001.

Katzenschlager, P., R. Fliedl, C. Popow, and M. Kundi. 2018. "Quality of life and satisfaction with inpatient treatment in adolescents with psychiatric disorders A comparison between 'patients', parents', and 'caregivers' (self-)assessments at admission and discharge." *Neuropsychiatrie* 32 (2):75-83. doi: 10.1007/s40211-018-0264-3.

Kazdin, A. E., L. Holland, and M. Crowley. 1997. "Family experience of barriers to treatment and premature termination from child therapy." *Journal of Consulting and Clinical Psychology* 65 (3):453-463. doi: 10.1037/0022-006x.65.3.453.

Kazdin, A. E., and G. Wassell. 2000. "Predictors of Barriers to Treatment and Therapeutic Change in Outpatient Therapy for Antisocial Children and Their Families." *Mental Health Services Research* 1:27.40. doi: 10.1023/A:1010191807861.

Larsen, D. L., C. C. Attkisson, W. A. Hargreaves, and T. D. Nguyen. 1979. "Assessment of client/patient satisfaction: development of a general scale." *Eval Program Plann*: 197-207.

Lindstedt, K., L. Kjellin, and S. A. Gustafsson. 2017. "Adolescents with full or subthreshold anorexia nervosa in a naturalistic sample - characteristics and treatment outcome." *Journal of Eating Disorders* 5. doi: 10.1186/s40337-017-0135-5.

Madan, A., C. Sharp, E. Newlin, S. Vanwoerden, and J. C. Fowler. 2016. "Adolescents Are Less Satisfied with Inpatient Psychiatric Care than Their Parents: Does It Matter?" *Journal for Healthcare Quality* 38 (4):E19-E28. doi: 10.1111/jhq.12081.

Man, J., and M. Kangas. 2019. "Service satisfaction and helpfulness ratings, mental health literacy and help seeking barriers of carers of individuals with dual disabilities." *Journal of Applied Research in Intellectual Disabilities* 32 (1):184-193. doi: 10.1111/jar.12520.

Mathiesen, S. G., S. J. Cash, and W. W. Hudson. 2002. "The multidimensional adolescent assessment scale: A validation study." *Research on Social Work Practice* 12 (1):9-28. doi: 10.1177/104973150201200103.

Mill, J. S. 1863. *Utilitarism*. London: Longman, Green, Longman, Roberst & Green.

Persson, S., C. Hagquist, and D. Michelson. 2017. "Young voices in mental health care: Exploring children's and adolescents' service experiences and preferences." *Clinical Child Psychology and Psychiatry* 22 (1):140-151. doi: 10.1177/1359104516656722.

Reardon, T., K. Harvey, M. Baranowska, D. O'Brien, L. Smith, and C. Creswell. 2017. "What do parents perceive are the barriers and facilitators to accessing psychological treatment for mental health problems in children and adolescents? A systematic review of qualitative and quantitative studies." *European Child & Adolescent Psychiatry* 26 (6):623-647. doi: 10.1007/s00787-016-0930-6.

Rey, J. M., J. M. Plapp, and P. L. Simpson. 1999. "Parental satisfaction and outcome: a 4-year study in a child and adolescent mental health service." *Australian and New Zealand Journal of Psychiatry* 33 (1):22-28. doi: 10.1046/j.1440-1614.1999.00516.x.

Ruggeri, M, R Dall'Agnola, G Bisoffi, and T. Greenfield. 1996. "Factor analysis of the Verona Service Satisfaction Scale-82 and devel-opment of reduced versions." *International Methods in Psychiatry Research* 6:23-38.

Sackett, D. L., W. M. Rosenberg, J. A. Gray, R. B. Haynes, and W. S. Richardson. 1996. "Evidence based medicine: what it is and what it isn't." *Bmj* 312 (7023):71-2. doi: 10.1136/bmj.312.7023.71.

Shirk, S. R., and M. Karver. 2003. "Prediction of treatment outcome from relationship variables in child and adolescent therapy: A meta-analytic review." *Journal of Consulting and Clinical Psychology* 71 (3):452-464. doi: 10.1037/0022-006x.71.3.452.

Stacey, K., S. Allison, V. Dadds, L. Roeger, A. Wood, and G. Martin. 2002. "The Relationship between Change and Satisfaction: Parents' Experiences in a Child and Adolescent Mental Health Service." *Australian and New Zealand Journal of Family Therapy* 23:79-89. doi: 10.1002/j.1467-8438.2002.tb00492.x.

Tas, F. V., T. Guvenir, and E. Cevrim. 2010. "Patients' and their parents' satisfaction levels about the treatment in a child and adolescent mental health inpatient unit." *Journal of Psychiatric and Mental Health Nursing* 17 (9):769-774. doi: 10.1111/j.1365-2850.2010.01612.x.

Urben, S., A. Gloor, V. Baier, G. Mantzouranis, C. Graap, M. Cherix-Parchet, C. Henz, F. Dutoit, A. Faucherand, E. Senent, and L. Holzer. 2015. "Patients' satisfaction with community treatment: a pilot cross-sectional survey adopting multiple perspectives." *Journal of Psychiatric and Mental Health Nursing* 22 (9):680-687. doi: 10.1111/jpm.12240.

Viefhaus, P., M. Dopfner, L. Dachs, H. Goletz, A. Gortz-Dorten, C. Kinnen, D. Perri, C. Rademacher, S. Schurmann, K. Woitecki, T. W. Metternich-Kaizman, and D. Walter. 2019. "Treatment satisfaction following routine outpatient cognitive-behavioral therapy of adolescents with mental disorders: a triple perspective of patients, parents and therapists." *European Child & Adolescent Psychiatry* 28 (4):543-556. doi: 10.1007/s00787-018-1220-2.

Viefhaus, P., M. Dopfner, L. Dachs, H. Goletz, A. Gortz-Dorten, C. Kinnen, D. Perri, C. Rademacher, S. Schurmann, K. Woitecki, T. W. Metternich-Kaizman, and D. Walter. 2020. "Parent- and therapist-rated treatment satisfaction following routine child cognitive-behavioral therapy." *European Child & Adolescent Psychiatry*. doi: 10.1007/s00787-020-01528-1.

Vusio, F., A. Thompson, M. Birchwood, and L. Clarke. 2019. "Experiences and satisfaction of children, young people and their parents with alternative mental health models to inpatient settings: a systematic review." *European Child & Adolescent Psychiatry*. doi: 10.1007/s00787-019-01420-7.

WHO. 2013. *Mental health action plan 2013-2020.* https://www.who.int/mental_health/action_plan_2013/mhap_brochure.pdf.

WHO. 2019. "10 facts on mental health." https://www.who.int/news-room/facts-in-pictures/detail/mental-health.

Widmark, C., C. Sandahl, K. Piuva, and D. Bergman. 2013. "Parents' experiences of collaboration between welfare professionals regarding children with anxiety or depression - an explorative study." *International Journal of Integrated Care* 13.

Wisdom, J. P., M. Cavaleri, L. Gogel, and M. Nacht. 2011. "Barriers and facilitators to adolescent drug treatment: Youth, family, and staff reports." *Addiction Research & Theory* 19 (2):179-188. doi: 10.3109/16066359.2010.530711.

Yalom, I. D. 1980. *Existential Psychotherapy*. New York, NY, US: Basic Books.

Zaitsoff, S. L., and A. Taylor. 2009. "Factors Related to Motivation for Change in Adolescents with Eating Disorders." *European Eating Disorders Review* 17 (3):227-233. doi: 10.1002/erv.915.

In: Patient Satisfaction
Editor: Dielle Morneau
ISBN: 978-1-53618-613-0
© 2020 Nova Science Publishers, Inc.

Chapter 3

BREAST RECONSTRUCTION: A REVIEW OF FACTORS AFFECTING PATIENT SATISFACTION AND QUALITY OF LIFE

Maleka Ramji and Farrah Yau
Division of Plastic Surgery, University of Calgary
Calgary, Alberta, Canada

ABSTRACT

Breast cancer is the most common cancer affecting women worldwide, with one in eight females diagnosed before the age of 85 years. Many survivors are young and live on for decades following treatment with 5-year survival rates as high as 90%.

Oncologic management of breast cancer includes lumpectomy with adjuvant radiation or mastectomy alone. This choice is impacted by a myriad of factors, relying on a shared decision-making process between the breast surgeon and patient. Over the years, we have seen an increasing trend for mastectomy, which often has a significant impact on a woman's quality of life, body image and sexuality. For decades, breast reconstruction, both autologous and alloplastic has been relied upon to address these concerns and impart a sense of 'wholeness' for women.

Reconstruction also allows women to limit their use of external prosthesis and wear a greater variety of clothing.

There are many factors that impact patient satisfaction and quality of life, following breast reconstruction. This chapter will explore and review current literature on what these factors are and their impact on patient quality of life. With health-related quality of life (HRQoL) central to the success of breast reconstruction, the study and measurement of patient reported outcomes (PROs) has allowed surgeons to evaluate these factors with greater thoughtfulness. Assessment tools such as the BREAST-Q have been designed for evaluating outcomes in breast reconstruction and remains the most frequently used validated breast reconstructive questionnaire.

Several surgical factors have been identified as being key players impacting patient reported outcomes. These include the type of reconstruction performed (autologous versus alloplastic and the type of implant used), the timing of the reconstruction and whether surgery is unilateral or bilateral. Additional factors have also been distilled that have received increased attention in recent years. These include clinical variables, psychosocial variables and sociodemographic variables. Understanding these factors is vitally important for surgeons performing breast reconstructive procedures, to enhance quality of care, address patient's expectations and optimize future breast surgery research.

INTRODUCTION

Breast cancer is the most common malignancy affecting women worldwide. While oncologic management could include lumpectomy with adjuvant radiation or mastectomy alone, we have seen an increasing trend towards mastectomy in recent years [1]. Survival rates are favorable, making women with a history of breast cancer the largest group of cancer survivors worldwide [2]. This reality has placed an increased focus on minimizing the morbidity of mastectomy surgery, which can lead to a range of long term psychosocial sequalae. Improving the quality of life of women through breast reconstruction has been advocated to impart a greater sense of self-esteem and body image as well as improve psychological and sexual satisfaction.

Breast reconstruction can be performed through various means. Options include breast implants, local flaps, free flaps, fat grafting or a combination of multiple modalities. Breast implants, since their introduction into the market in the 1960's have undergone many iterations and today have a more natural feel, with lesser incidence of capsular contracture [3]. Generally, this reconstructive option is common in young women with non-irradiated chests who are seeking a shorter post-operative recovery and hospital stay. There have also been stark advancements in microsurgical techniques in the last two decades. This has lent to the development of a variety of free flap options, including tissue from the abdomen, buttock, low back, and inner thigh. Furthermore, abdominal based options have become more sophisticated and include muscle sparing and single perforator techniques with decreased donor site morbidity.

The primary goal of breast reconstruction is to improve a woman's body image and sense of self. The patient's perception of the aesthetics, look and feel of their breasts has a direct impact on their sense of physical and psychosocial wellbeing. It is therefore of utmost importance that the surgeon understands the desire and expectations of the patient to provide a satisfying result [4]. Patient reported outcomes (PRO) research, is of crucial importance to achieve this. In addition, assessment tools such as the BREAST-Q have been designed to evaluate outcomes in breast reconstruction and remains the most frequently used and validated breast reconstructive questionnaire.

Patient Reported Outcome Tools

The Breast-Q was developed by a group of surgeons to address the lack of existing breast surgery-related outcome measurement tools, specifically in the domain of patient reported outcomes. A systematic review conducted by *Pusic* et al. identified 227 health outcome questionnaires used in previous breast surgery studies. However, there was only one measure known as the Breast-Related Symptoms Questionnaire that had adequate development and validation in the target population [5]. Unfortunately, this tool was marred with substantial content limitations. As such, the BREAST-Q was developed and validated, with adherence to best practice guidelines, robust in depth patient and clinician interviews, literature reviews, focus groups and clinician interviews. The BREAST-Q includes 5 modules: (1) Augmentation, (2) Reduction/Mastopexy, (3) Mastectomy, (4) Reconstruction and (5) Breast Conserving Therapy. Each module covers two categories for both the pre and post-operative stages: health related quality of life outcomes (HR-QOL) and patient satisfaction. The BREAST-Q answers are imputed and scored using an executable software application called Q-score. The program then estimates a Rasch-based person measure, ranging from 0 to 100, which is based on a calibration of each set of items in each scale [6]. A higher BREAST-Q score means better HR-QoL or greater satisfaction.

Other PRO tools are often applied in research studies. Most commonly seen are the 36 Item Short Form Survey (SF-36) and the European Organization for Research and Treatment of Cancer (EORTC) Breast Cancer-Specific Quality of Life Questionnaire (QLQ-BR23). The SF-36 is a generic, easy to administer quality of life survey conducted by the RAND Corporation [7]. The SF-36 consists of eight scaled scores, including (1) vitality, (2) physical functioning, (3) bodily pain, (4) general health perceptions, (5) physical role functioning, (6) emotional role functioning, (7) social role functioning, and (8) mental health [8]. Each scale is transformed into a 0-100 scale with higher scores, reflecting less disability [9]. This scale has not been validated for use in breast cancer or breast reconstruction. By contrast, the EORTC QLQBR23 is a core cancer-specific quality of life questionnaire, with a specific breast cancer instrument. It has 23 items, with two functional scales (body image and sexual functioning) and three symptoms scales (arm symptoms, breast symptoms and systematic therapy side effects) [10]. This tool has undergone a few iterations, and was recently updated to include 22 additional items. It is currently in phase 4 of testing to assess psychometric properties and validity in patients diagnosed with breast cancer at various stages of treatment [11].

Several surgical factors have been identified as key items impacting patient reported outcomes. These include the type of reconstruction performed (autologous versus alloplastic), the timing of the reconstruction, whether surgery is unilateral or bilateral and the implant choice of saline versus silicone. Additional non-surgical factors have also been explored and include clinical, psychosocial and sociodemographic factors. Understanding these factors and their impact on patient satisfaction and quality of life scores is vitally important for surgeons performing breast reconstructive procedures.

SUGRICAL VARIABLES

Unilateral versus Bilateral Mastectomy and Reconstruction

Bilateral mastectomy in breast cancer patients increased three-fold from 2005 to 2012, which also resulted in an increase in bilateral reconstruction rates [12]. This may be partly due to an increasing number of unilateral breast cancer patients who are exploring the merit of contralateral prophylactic mastectomy and simultaneous reconstruction. Women who are genetic carriers, specifically BRAC1/2, are also seeking prophylactic bilateral mastectomies and subsequent immediate bilateral breast reconstruction [13].

Kuykendall et al. evaluated patient reported outcomes in patients undergoing unilateral versus bilateral breast reconstruction with either DIEP flap autologous reconstruction or implant-based reconstruction. They found that patients undergoing unilateral breast reconstruction demonstrated higher satisfaction in the categories of psychosocial and sexual well-being when compared to the bilateral reconstruction group. With consideration of reconstructive type, patients who underwent DIEP flap reconstruction demonstrated higher satisfaction with unilateral reconstruction. They postulated that bilateral reconstruction may not provide adequate volume to replicate both missing breasts, leading to poorer aesthetic outcome and potential for greater donor site morbidity. Those patients who underwent implant based reconstruction, demonstrated no significant difference in satisfaction scores between unilateral and bilateral reconstruction [14].

Patients were evaluated for the same clinical question in a multicenter prospective cohort study by *Taylor* et al., *where patients were recruited over a 5 year period*. Patients were captured through the Mastectomy Reconstruction Outcomes Consortium (MROC). Of 2125 patients, 917 (43%) underwent unilateral breast reconstruction and 1208 (57%) underwent bilateral breast reconstruction [15]. Patient reported outcome measures (PROM) were assessed through the BREAST-Q breast reconstruction module. In the setting of unilateral breast reconstruction, autologous flap reconstruction was associated with higher satisfaction rates when compared to implant-based reconstruction. Similarly, for bilateral reconstruction, the autologous group also had higher satisfaction rates when compared to implant-based reconstruction, but their scores were reduced by approximately 50 percent compared to the unilateral cohort.

In summary, for patients who opted for autologous reconstruction, better satisfaction rates were obtained in those who selected unilateral over bilateral reconstruction. For patients who opted for implant reconstruction, there was no difference in satisfaction between unilateral and bilateral reconstruction. In addition, regardless of whether the reconstruction was unilateral or bilateral, patients were more satisfied with autologous reconstruction.

Timing of Reconstruction

The goal of the surgical treatment of breast cancer is to achieve local cure with complete excision of disease and minimization of the risk of recurrence [16]. As a result, when immediate breast reconstruction (IBR) was introduced as a method to minimize patient morbidity, concerns with regards to oncologic outcomes surfaced. Oncologists and surgeons worried that IBR could delay the delivery of adjuvant therapies and the detection of recurrence.

Numerous studies have since been conducted to address these oncologic considerations. The literature is abundant in demonstrating that the incidence of local recurrence after mastectomy alone is comparable to local recurrence after immediate breast reconstruction (IBR) [17 18]. A systematic review on the topic conducted in 2012 by *Gieni* et al., found that local recurrence rates were not higher in patients that underwent IBR and that there was no increase in systemic recurrence [16]. A prospective, multicenter cohort study, recruiting 2652 patients, assessed whether IBR influenced the time to delivery of adjuvant therapy compared with mastectomy alone. Their study found that IBR did not result in clinically significant delays of adjuvant treatment compared to mastectomy alone. However, they did find that complications, particularly those requiring repeat surgery or hospital admission, did result in a significant delay of either chemotherapy or radiation. Essentially, it was post-operative complications, rather than procedure type, that served as the main predictor of adjuvant treatment delay [19 20]. In recent years, IBR has become the preferred option for reconstruction among surgeons in the USA. This approach has been supported as it is thought to result in lower hospital costs, improved breast reconstructive aesthetics and better psychosocial and physical well-being for patients [21].

A cross-sectional survey study by *Beugels* et al. evaluated patients by way of the BREAST-Q at a single time stamp 12 months post-operatively. They found that patients reported equal quality of life scores with both immediate and delayed DIEP flap reconstruction following mastectomy [22]. Similar findings were noted by *Yoon* et al. in a multi-center prospective cohort study evaluating PROs at 2 years post-operatively. Reconstruction procedure types included direct-to-implant, tissue expanders/implant and various pedicled and free flap autologous procedures. Again, timing of reconstruction was found to have no significant effect on PROs. Both immediate and delayed cohort's unadjusted and adjusted BREAST-Q, PROMIC and EORTC-QLQ-BR23 subscale scores, showed no statistically significant differences [23]. One notable difference however, was the pre-operative PROs score between the two cohorts. The cohort that underwent delayed reconstruction had lower levels of psychosocial, physical, and sexual well-being when compared to the group that underwent immediate reconstruction. This difference highlights the impact of mastectomy alone on the mental and physical wellbeing of women. Similar findings were reported by *Domenico* et al. who compared immediate versus delayed breast reconstruction groups using the BREAST-Q. They found that patients undergoing delayed reconstruction had significantly lower Q-scores in quality of life domains pre-operatively, when compared to the immediate reconstruction cohort. However, at 12 months following reconstruction, the immediate and delayed group had no differences in quality of life domains [24]. Taking into consideration these low pre-operative well-being scores, immediate reconstruction may appear to be the obvious choice for treatment timing. However, it may not the most suitable course of treatment for all women; the timing of treatment should be considered on a case by case basis. Some women who are known to require post-operative radiation, for example, may be better suited for delayed reconstruction to avoid potential complications that could delay adjuvant therapy. In addition, those women with significant medical comorbidities may not be able to tolerate the longer operating times associated with immediate reconstruction.

Ultimately, both immediate and delayed breast reconstruction provide significant quality of life benefits to the patient; the choice regarding the timing of reconstruction should be discussed in detail with the patient and tailored to their specific needs. Reassuringly, women who opt to postpone reconstruction for oncologic, medical or personal preferences, will not miss out on the ultimate quality of life impact when compared to those who opt for immediate reconstruction.

Implant versus Autologous Reconstruction

The decision of whether to undergo implant or autologous based reconstruction is a key consideration in breast reconstruction. Many factors influence this decision, including patient age, donor site availability, oncological disease characteristics and surgeon preference. Several studies have assessed patient satisfaction and PROs when comparing these two interventions. The BREAST-Q has been utilized as the central validated assessment tool.

At one year following immediate breast reconstruction, one study found that those patients who underwent autologous reconstruction were more satisfied with their breasts and had greater psychosocial and sexual well-being than did patients who underwent implant reconstruction. There was however, no difference in physical well-being between these two groups [25].

A multicenter prospective trial, recruiting patients from the North American Mastectomy Reconstruction Outcomes Consortium (MROC) evaluated patient reported outcomes, specifically with regards to autologous versus alloplastic reconstruction with a minimum of 2-years follow-up. Once again, those who underwent autologous reconstruction reported significantly higher levels of satisfaction with their breasts and quality of life (QoL), as measured by higher psychosocial, physical, and sexual wellbeing scores, than those who underwent alloplastic reconstruction. However, the donor site morbidity associated with autologous reconstruction should be considered. While breast scores are superior for autologous reconstructive patients, donor site morbidity did contribute to lower scores. Abdominal well-being amongst patients who underwent abdominal based reconstruction worsened from baseline in the first post-operative year, and continued to be inferior even at two years post-operatively. The difference was significant with a mean decrease of thirteen points in the physical well-being of the abdomen score, two years post-operatively [26]. Therefore, although breast satisfaction is higher than alloplastic reconstruction in these patients, the donor site morbidity is considerable and does significantly lower physical well-being scores.

More recently, a systematic review strictly comparing quality of life outcomes and cost-effectiveness between DIEP and implant-based breast reconstruction, identified two comparative studies evaluating QoL. *Matros* et al. prospectively evaluated 103 patients with DIEP-based breast reconstruction and 172 patients with implant-based reconstruction. Once again, BREAST-Q scores were consistently higher for DIEP-reconstructed patients compared with implant-reconstructed patients post-operatively, with the longest follow-up at eight years [27]. *Tosenth* et al. analysed the same clinical outcomes, using instead the generic PRO tool, the short form

36 (SF-36). Interestingly, and converse to the above findings, SF-36 found no difference in quality of life, between implant versus autologous based reconstruction [28].

With application of the BREAST-Q, both a multi-center prospective trial and systematic review of available literature suggested that autologous based breast reconstruction yields higher patient satisfaction than alloplastic reconstruction. In spite of this, patients should always be informed of both options and specifically counselled on the impact of donor site morbidity with autologous reconstruction. Of additional importance, are the differences between the length of recovery and the complication profile of alloplastic versus autologous reconstruction [29]. These differences might sway a patient to choose one treatment over the other, and therefore the choice of reconstruction should be tailored to each patient's specific needs.

Saline versus Silicone Implant-Based Reconstruction

The debate between silicone versus saline implant reconstruction has long prevailed in the plastic surgery community. A multicenter cross-sectional study was performed over a 20-month period to capture predictors of satisfaction including breast appearance and implant type, in women who underwent post-mastectomy implant-based reconstruction. A questionnaire, containing the BREAST-Q was distributed to eligible patients and the response rate was 77% [30]. Specific to implant material choice, women with silicone-based reconstruction reported higher levels of satisfaction than those with saline based reconstruction [30].

Corroborating these findings, a smaller cross-sectional study was performed in a single center with patient reported outcome measures captured using the BREAST-Q and the EORTC QLQC30. The response rate for silicone and saline implant recipients was 75% and 58%, respectively. Mean scores were compared between silicone and saline recipients. Silicone implant recipients once again scored higher on all nine subscales within the BREAST-Q. The subscales included (1) satisfaction with breast, (2) satisfaction with outcome, (3) psychological well-being, (4) sexual well-being, (5) physical well-being, (6) satisfaction with information, (7) satisfaction with surgeon, (8) satisfaction with medical staff and (9) satisfaction with office staff. This difference reached statistical significance for only four of the nine subscales, which included satisfaction with breast, psychological well-being, satisfaction with surgeon and sexual well-being. Multi-variable linear regression analysis showed a statistically significant association between silicone implant recipients and high scores in the same four BREAST-Q subscales [31]. Scores using the EORTC QLQ30, did not differ as significantly between the saline and silicone implant recipients. Only with regards to physical function, did silicone patients have higher overall scores [31].

The findings above support previously held opinions regarding implant-breast reconstruction. Anecdotally, many surgeons believe that silicone gel implants provide a more natural appearing and feeling result, when compared with saline implant reconstruction and the same is confirmed by breast reconstructive patients.

ADDITIONAL/NON-SURGICAL VARIABLES

Psychosocial Variables

As highlighted by the findings of the BREAST-Q, breast reconstruction is associated with psychological benefits including improved body image, self-esteem, and mood [32]. These benefits are captured in various scenarios, including both immediate and delayed reconstruction as well as autologous and alloplastic reconstruction. Some studies, however, report similar patient reported outcomes following breast reconstruction even when compared to breast conservation surgery or mastectomy alone [33]. In fact, one study found poorer psychosocial functioning and increased mood disturbance in patients who underwent reconstruction compared to those with mastectomy alone [34]. These surprising and inconsistent patient reported outcomes have led researchers to consider what other variables may be responsible for patient satisfaction and quality of life.

Matthews et al. sought to clarify this in a cross-sectional retrospective study, evaluating the responses of one hundred and eighty women. They found that women with greater pre-operative psychological wellbeing were more likely to report greater satisfaction with breast appearance and outcome post- reconstruction [35]. Similarly, patients who underwent breast reconstruction with pre-operative symptoms of depression were more likely to have lower body self-image and quality of life scores post-operatively [36].

The impact of personality traits on quality of life outcomes, has also been evaluated in the breast reconstruction literature. *Juhl* et al., evaluated participating patients with the Neuroticism-Extraversion-Openness Five Factor Inventory (NEO-FFI) 60 item questionnaire. This tool identifies the five personality traits of neuroticism, extraversion, openness, agreeableness and conscientiousness. Neurotocism was found to be a statistically independent predictor of poorer quality of life and body image from baseline, at 6 months post-operatively [37]. Of note, neuroticism is a trait more commonly seen in anxious, self-conscious, stress-susceptible individuals with poor coping mechanisms [38]. *Juhl* et al. suggested that patients with this trait should not be dissuaded from breast reconstruction. Rather, these patients could be identified early and provided psychosocial support to help manage stress and improve coping mechanisms, with the potential opportunity to improve quality of life post-operatively [37].

Clinical Variables

The most significant clinical variables affecting quality of life following breast reconstruction, are body mass index (BMI) and the need for adjuvant therapies, as evidenced by the literature.

It is well established that breast reconstruction in overweight patients poses additional challenges, with an increased risk of complications and poorer aesthetic outcomes. Regarding implant-based reconstruction, *Fee-*

Fulkerson et al. found that patients with a higher BMI reported lower levels of satisfaction compared to women with a normal BMI [39].

Atisha et al. made differing conclusions based on reconstructive type. Patient BMI did not have a significant effect on general satisfaction for either autologous or alloplastic reconstruction. However, they found that with regards to aesthetic satisfaction, obese patients with expander/implant reconstructions were significantly less likely to be satisfied compared with patients with a normal BMI. For TRAM flaps, they found that BMI did not have a significant effect on aesthetic satisfaction. The authors posit that greater aesthetic satisfaction with TRAM flap reconstruction versus implant reconstruction in high BMI patients may be due to the better ability of autologous tissue to match a contralateral large volume, ptotic breast. It is also well established that autologous reconstruction generally yields increased patient satisfaction over alloplastic reconstruction, irrespective of BMI [40].

Unsurprisingly, adjuvant interventions can also impact quality of life scores in breast reconstructive patients. Radiation therapy is associated with a higher incidence of complications and poorer aesthetic outcomes. In a study by Devulapelli et al., at one-year follow-up, the non-irradiated group reported higher BREAST-Q scores when compared to the irradiated group, with regards to satisfaction with breasts, psychosocial well-being, sexual well-being, physical well-being of the chest, and satisfaction with outcome. When comparing irradiation in patients with alloplastic and autologous reconstruction, satisfaction with breasts and physical well-being of chest scores were initially worse in patients with alloplastic reconstruction [41]. However, at 1 year follow-up, these scores were comparable [41]. This finding provides support for implant-based reconstruction even in irradiated patients. Recent advancements with the use of acellular dermal matrices and fat grafting have let to improved late aesthetic outcomes in the irradiated alloplastic reconstructive cohort.

Sociodemographic Variables

Quality of life is a multi-dimensional entity referring to a combination of physical, psychological, social, and spiritual domains. Age, marital status, education level and work status are the sociodemographic characteristics that have shown to impact quality of life following breast reconstruction [42].

Advanced age is a common feature among women diagnosed with breast cancer. According to the Surveillance, Epidemiology and End Results Database, in 2016, of the nearly 250 000 women diagnosed with breast cancer, forty percent of them were over the age or 62 years [43]. Despite this, older women are less likely than their younger counterparts to undergo reconstructive surgery following mastectomy. Surgeons may be less likely to offer interventions to the older patient due to concerns of increased complications. In addition, older women themselves may be fearful of surgical interventions and cannot justify the benefits over the potential risks [44].

A large, prospective, multicenter study conducted by *Santosa* et al. sought to analyze the impact that age has on quality of life outcomes in breast reconstructive patients. Women were categorized by age group: 494 were less than age 45, 803 were between 45 and 60 years of age and 234 were over age 60. All were assessed via the BREAST-Q. Almost all groups of women, regardless of age, were just as satisfied with their breasts after reconstruction as pre-operatively. Only older women who specifically had implant-based reconstruction had a slight drop in the BREAST-Q satisfaction score from 60.9 preoperatively to 59.2 afterwards. This may be related to the known higher satisfaction scores of autologous over alloplastic reconstruction, independent of age [44].

CONCLUSION

The evaluation of patient satisfaction and quality of life following surgical intervention is a task of great importance and can provide us with information to best deliver optimal care to patients. Breast reconstruction, as a quality of life intervention, requires thoughtful evaluation of both the surgical and non-surgical variables that impact patient satisfaction. Existing research demonstrates some trends that support autologous reconstruction over alloplastic reconstruction and silicone over saline implants. However, clinical, psychosocial, and sociodemographic factors can lead to variability in patient satisfaction scores.

This reality behooves the surgeon to identify and best address individual patient needs and expectations as well as to educate and empower patients to be active in their own care. Efforts to design and conduct prospective studies should continue and include evaluating patient satisfaction relating to patient characteristics, identifying those patients at risk of dissatisfaction and assessing those interventions of greatest impact. Only in this way, can we continue to improve long-term post-operative satisfaction and quality life for this large cohort of breast reconstructive patients [45].

REFERENCES

[1] McGuire, KP; Santillan, AA; Kaur, P; et al. Are mastectomies on the rise? *A 13-year trend analysis of the selection of mastectomy versus breast conservation therapy in 5865 patients.*, 2009, 16(10), 2682-90.

[2] The changing face of cancer survivorship. *Seminars in Oncology Nursing*, 2001. Elsevier.

[3] Henderson, PW; Nash, D; Laskowski, M. Grant RTJAps. *Objective comparison of commercially available breast implant devices.*, 2015, 39(5), 724-32.

[4] Liu, LQ; Branford, OA; Mehigan, S. BREAST-Q Measurement of the Patient Perspective in Oncoplastic Breast Surgery: A Systematic Review. Plastic and reconstructive surgery. *Global open*, 2018, 6(8), e1904 doi: https://dx.doi.org/10.1097/GOX.0000000000001904 [published Online First: Epub Date]|.

[5] Pusic, AL; Chen, CM; Cano, S; et al. *Measuring quality of life in cosmetic and reconstructive breast surgery: a systematic review of patient-reported outcomes instruments.*, 2007, 120(4), 823-37.

[6] Cano, SJ; Klassen, AF; Scott, AM; Pusic, AL. A closer look at the BREAST-Q(©). *Clinics in plastic surgery*, 2013, 40(2), 287-96 doi: https://dx.doi.org/10.1016/j.cps.2012.12.002 [published Online First: Epub Date]|.

[7] *36-Item Short Form Survey from the RAND Medical Outcomes Study.* Secondary "36-Item Short Form Survey from the RAND Medical Outcomes Study." www.rand.org/health-care/surveys_tools/ mos/36-item-short-form.html.

[8] Ware, Jr JE; Sherbourne, CDJMc. The MOS 36-item short-form health survey (SF-36): I. *Conceptual framework and item selection.*, 1992, 473-83.

[9] Treanor, C; Donnelly, MJQolr. *A methodological review of the Short Form Health Survey 36 (SF-36) and its derivatives among breast cancer survivors.*, 2015, 24(2), 339-62.

[10] Cordova, LZ; Hunter-Smith, DJ; Rozen, WM. Patient reported outcome measures (PROMs) following mastectomy with breast reconstruction or without reconstruction: a systematic review. *Gland surgery*, 2019, 8(4), 441-51 doi: https://dx.doi.org/10.21037/gs.2019.07.02 [published Online First: Epub Date]|.

[11] Bjelic-Radisic, V. "Breast Cancer (Update of QLQ-BR23): EORTC – Quality of Life." *Secondary "Breast Cancer (Update of QLQ-BR23): EORTC – Quality of Life.,"* 15 Oct, 2019. qol.eortc.org/questionnaire/update-qlq-br23/.

[12] Kwok, AC; Goodwin, IA; Ying, J; Agarwal, JPJTAJoS. *National trends and complication rates after bilateral mastectomy and immediate breast reconstruction from 2005 to 2012.*, 2015, 210(3), 512-16.

[13] Franceschini, G; Di Leone, A; Terribile, D; Sanchez, MA; Masetti, R. *Bilateral prophylactic mastectomy in BRCA mutation carriers: what surgeons need to know*, 2019.

[14] Kuykendall, LV; Tugertimur, B; Agoris, C; Bijan, S; Kumar, A; Dayicioglu, D. Unilateral Versus Bilateral Breast Reconstruction: Is Less Really More? *Annals of plastic surgery*, 2017, 78, (6S Suppl 5), S275-S78 doi: https://dx.doi.org/10.1097/ SAP.0000000000001030 [published Online First: Epub Date]|.

[15] Taylor, EM; Wilkins, EG; Pusic, AL; et al. Impact of Unilateral versus Bilateral Breast Reconstruction on Procedure Choices and Outcomes. *Plastic and reconstructive surgery*, 2019, 143(6), 1159e-68e doi: https://dx.doi.org/10.1097/PRS.0000000000005602 [published Online First: Epub Date]|.

[16] Gieni, M; Avram, R; Dickson, L; et al. *Local breast cancer recurrence after mastectomy and immediate breast reconstruction for invasive cancer: a meta-analysis.*, 2012, 21(3), 230-36.

[17] Van Mierlo, D; Penha, TL; Schipper, R; et al. *No increase of local recurrence rate in breast cancer patients treated with skin-sparing mastectomy followed by immediate breast reconstruction.*, 2013, 22(6), 1166-70.

[18] Zhang, P; Li, CZ; Wu, CT; et al. *Comparison of immediate breast reconstruction after mastectomy and mastectomy alone for breast cancer: a meta-analysis.*, 2017, 43(2), 285-93.

[19] Riba, LA; Gruner, RA; Fleishman, A; James, TAJAoso. *Surgical risk factors for the delayed initiation of adjuvant chemotherapy in breast cancer.*, 2018, 25(7), 1904-11.

[20] O'Connell, RL; Rattay, T; Dave, RV; et al. *The impact of immediate breast reconstruction on the time to delivery of adjuvant therapy: the iBRA-2 study.*, 2019, 120(9), 883-95.

[21] Yoon, AP; Qi, J; Brown, DL; et al. Outcomes of immediate versus delayed breast reconstruction: Results of a multicenter prospective study. *Breast (Edinburgh, Scotland)*, 2018, 37(9213011), 72-79 doi: https://dx.doi.org/10.1016/j.breast.2017.10.009 [published Online First: Epub Date]|.

[22] Beugels, J; Kool, M; Hoekstra, LT; et al. Quality of Life of Patients After Immediate or Delayed Autologous Breast Reconstruction: A Multicenter Study. *Annals of plastic surgery*, 2018, 81(5), 523-27

doi: https://dx.doi.org/10.1097/SAP.0000000000001618[published Online First: Epub Date]|.

[23] Yoon, AP; Qi, J; Brown, DL; et al. *Outcomes of immediate versus delayed breast reconstruction: Results of a multicenter prospective study.*, 2018, 37, 72-79.

[24] Pagliara, D; Albanese, R; Storti, G; Adesi, LB; Salgarello, MJP; Open, RSG. *Patient-reported Outcomes in Immediate and Delayed Breast Reconstruction with Deep Inferior Epigastric Perforator Flap.*, 2018, 6(2).

[25] Pusic, AL; Matros, E; Fine, N; et al. Patient-Reported Outcomes 1 Year After Immediate Breast Reconstruction: Results of the Mastectomy Reconstruction Outcomes Consortium Study. *Journal of clinical oncology: official journal of the American Society of Clinical Oncology*, 2017, 35(22), 2499-506 doi: https://dx.doi.org/10.1200/JCO.2016.69.9561[published Online First: Epub Date]|.

[26] Santosa, KB; Qi, J; Kim, HM; Hamill, JB; Wilkins, EG; Pusic, AL. Long-term Patient-Reported Outcomes in Postmastectomy Breast Reconstruction. *JAMA surgery*, 2018, 153(10), 891-99 doi: https://dx.doi.org/10.1001/jamasurg.2018.1677 [published Online First: Epub Date]|.

[27] Matros, E; Albornoz, CR; Razdan, SN; et al. *Cost-effectiveness analysis of implants versus autologous perforator flaps using the BREAST-Q.*, 2015, 135(4), 937-46.

[28] Tønseth, K; Hokland, B; Tindholdt, T; Åbyholm, F. Stavem KJJop, reconstructive, surgery a. *Quality of life, patient satisfaction and cosmetic outcome after breast reconstruction using DIEP flap or expandable breast implant.*, 2008, 61(10), 1188-94.

[29] Pirro, O; Mestak, O; Vindigni, V; et al. Comparison of Patient-reported Outcomes after Implant Versus Autologous Tissue Breast Reconstruction Using the BREAST-Q. Plastic and reconstructive surgery. *Global open*, 2017, 5(1), e1217 doi: https://dx.doi.org/10.1097/GOX.0000000000001217 [published Online First: Epub Date]|.

[30] McCarthy, CM; Klassen, AF; Cano, SJ; et al. Patient satisfaction with postmastectomy breast reconstruction: a comparison of saline and silicone implants. *Cancer*, 2010, 116(24), 5584-91 doi: https://dx.doi.org/10.1002/cncr.25552 [published Online First: Epub Date]|.

[31] Macadam, SA; Ho, AL; Cook, EF; Jr. Lennox, PA; Pusic, AL. Patient satisfaction and health-related quality of life following breast reconstruction: patient-reported outcomes among saline and silicone implant recipients. *Plastic and reconstructive surgery*, 2010, 125(3), 761-71 doi: https://dx.doi.org/10.1097/ PRS.0b013e3181cb5cf8 [published Online First: Epub Date]|.

[32] Fingeret, MC; Nipomnick, SW; Crosby, MA; Reece, GP. Developing a theoretical framework to illustrate associations among patient satisfaction, body image and quality of life for women undergoing breast reconstruction. *Cancer treatment reviews*, 2013, 39(6), 673-81 doi: https://dx.doi.org/10.1016/j.ctrv.2012.12.010 [published Online First: Epub Date]|.

[33] Parker, PA; Youssef, A; Walker, S; et al. *Short-term and long-term psychosocial adjustment and quality of life in women undergoing different surgical procedures for breast cancer.*, 2007, 14(11), 3078-89.

[34] Nissen, MJ; Swenson, KK; Ritz, LJ; Farrell, JB; Sladek, ML; Lally, RMJC. *Quality of life after breast carcinoma surgery: a comparison of three surgical procedures.*, 2001, 91(7), 1238-46.

[35] Matthews, H; Carroll, N; Renshaw, D; et al. Predictors of satisfaction and quality of life following post-mastectomy breast reconstruction. *Psycho-oncology*, 2017, 26(11), 1860-65 doi: https://dx.doi.org/ 10.1002/pon.4397 [published Online First: Epub Date]|.

[36] Szadowska-Szlachetka, ZC; Stanislawek, A; Kachaniuk, H; et al. *Occurrence of depression symptoms measured by the Beck Depression Inventory (BDI) in women after mastectomy and breast reconstruction with regard to the assessment of quality of life.*, 2013, 12(4).

[37] Juhl, AA; Christensen, S; Zachariae, R; Damsgaard, TE. Unilateral breast reconstruction after mastectomy - patient satisfaction, aesthetic outcome and quality of life. *Acta oncologica* (Stockholm, Sweden), 2017, 56(2), 225-31 doi: https://dx.doi.org/10.1080/0284186X.2016.1266087 [published Online First: Epub Date]|.

[38] Costa, P; McCrae, R; Revised, NJPAR; Odessa, FL. *Personality Inventory (NEO-PI-R) and NEO Five-Factor Inventory (NEO-FFI): Professional Manual.*, 1992.

[39] Fee-Fulkerson, K; Conaway, MR; Winer, EP; et al. *Factors contributing to patient satisfaction with breast reconstruction using silicone gel implants.*, 1996, 97(7), 1420-26.

[40] Atisha, DM; Alderman, AK; Kuhn, LE; Wilkins, EG. The impact of obesity on patient satisfaction with breast reconstruction. *Plastic and Reconstructive Surgery*, 2008, 121(6), 1893-99 doi: http://dx.doi.org/10.1097/PRS.0b013e3181715198 [published Online First: Epub Date]|.

[41] Devulapalli, C; Bello, RJ; Moin, E; et al. The Effect of Radiation on Quality of Life throughout the Breast Reconstruction Process: A Prospective, Longitudinal Pilot Study of 200 Patients with Long-Term Follow-Up. *Plastic and reconstructive surgery*, 2018, 141(3), 579-89 doi: https://dx.doi.org/10.1097/PRS.0000000000004105 [published Online First: Epub Date]|.

[42] Sousa, H; Castro, S; Abreu, J; Pereira, MG. A systematic review of factors affecting quality of life after postmastectomy breast reconstruction in women with breast cancer. *Psycho-oncology*, 2019, 28(11), 2107-18 doi: https://dx.doi.org/10.1002/pon.5206 [published Online First: Epub Date]|.

[43] Howlader, N; Noone, A; Krapcho, M; et al. SEER *Cancer Statistics Review, 1975-2013*, National Cancer Institute. Bethesda, MD, 2016.

[44] Santosa, KB; Qi, J; Kim, HM; Hamill, JB; Pusic, AL; Wilkins, EG. Effect of Patient Age on Outcomes in Breast Reconstruction: Results from a Multicenter Prospective Study. *Journal of the American College of Surgeons*, 2016, 223(6), 745-54 doi: https://dx.doi.org/

10.1016/j.jamcollsurg.2016.09.003[published Online First: Epub Date]|.

[45] Pusic, AL; Klassen, AF; Snell, L; et al. Measuring and managing patient expectations for breast reconstruction: Impact on quality of life and patient satisfaction. *Expert Review of Pharmacoeconomics and Outcomes Research*, 2012, 12(2), 149-58 doi: http://dx.doi.org/10.1586/erp.11.105[published Online First: Epub Date]|.

INDEX

A

access to care, 6
adherence, 5, 11, 14, 21, 26, 27, 32, 34, 37, 39, 40, 41, 46, 50, 52, 54, 56, 58, 60, 62, 65, 101
adolescents, viii, 7, 67, 69, 70, 74, 75, 76, 95, 96, 97
advancements, 101, 111
adverse event, 10, 13
adverse events, 10, 13, 35, 63
aesthetic, 103, 110, 111, 118
age, viii, 69, 76, 79, 83, 84, 88, 99, 106, 112
alloplastic, ix, 99, 100, 102, 107, 108, 109, 111, 112, 113
anesthesia, 18, 25, 48, 49, 55
anesthesiology, 15
anorexia nervosa, 95
antisocial behavior, 75
anxiety, 8, 22, 35, 43, 52, 61, 64, 70, 75, 90, 97
assessment, vii, 77, 83, 88, 93, 101, 106, 117
assessment tools, vii, 101
asthma, 5, 6, 26, 27, 30, 54

autologous, ix, 99, 100, 102, 103, 104, 105, 106, 107, 108, 109, 111, 112, 113, 115, 116
awareness, 15, 79, 84

B

back pain, 8, 9
behaviors, 18, 75, 76, 81
benefits, 7, 11, 106, 109, 112
bilateral, ix, 100, 103, 104, 114
boarding, 12, 23
body image, ix, 82, 87, 99, 100, 101, 102, 109, 110, 117
body mass index, 110
breast cancer, viii, 19, 99, 100, 102, 103, 104, 112, 114, 115, 117, 118
breast carcinoma, 117
breast reconstruction, iv, v, vii, ix, 99, 100, 101, 102, 103, 104, 105, 106, 107, 108, 109, 110, 112, 113, 114, 115, 116, 117, 118, 119
breast surgery, ix, 15, 100, 101, 113, 114

BREAST-Q, iv, vii, ix, 100, 101, 104, 105, 106, 107, 108, 109, 111, 112, 113, 114, 116

C

cancer, viii, 5, 7, 14, 18, 19, 20, 21, 22, 25, 29, 31, 39, 40, 44, 46, 54, 55, 59, 61, 63, 64, 99, 100, 102, 103, 104, 112, 113, 114, 115, 117, 118
cancer care, 19
cancer screening, 5, 22, 31, 54
cardiac surgery, 14
cardiovascular disease, 5, 7, 21, 53
celiac disease, 21, 37
challenges, 91, 110
chemotherapy, 105, 115
child and adolescent mental health service, 68, 69, 92, 94, 96
Child and Adolescent Mental Health Service (CAMHS), v, viii, 67, 69, 70, 71, 72, 74, 75, 76, 77, 88, 89, 92, 93, 96
children, viii, 67, 69, 70, 74, 76, 77, 80, 82, 84, 86, 89, 93, 96, 97
chronic obstructive pulmonary disease, 7, 30
chronic pain, 8, 22, 25, 38, 49, 59
clinical oncology, 116
cognitive-behavioral therapy, 97
collaboration, 4, 69, 78, 89, 90, 97
colon cancer, 19
communication, vii, 1, 4, 5, 6, 8, 9, 11, 16, 18, 21, 22, 23, 24, 31, 32, 33, 37, 38, 40, 46, 50, 52, 53, 54, 55, 58, 61, 63, 65, 73, 76, 78, 82, 85, 89, 90
community, 69, 80, 97, 108
complexity, 71, 90, 91
complications, 14, 15, 16, 17, 18, 23, 28, 30, 105, 106, 110, 111, 112
congestive heart failure, 7, 10
conscientiousness, 110
conservation, 109, 113
correlation, 6, 8, 11, 16, 19, 23
cosmetic, 18, 114, 116
cost, 3, 15, 17, 23, 31, 37, 39, 51, 78, 87, 107, 116
critical care, 11, 13
cross-sectional study, 108
crowding, 12, 23, 27, 28, 41, 42, 50, 54, 55, 58

D

decision-making process, viii, 99
decubitus ulcer, 10
depression, 9, 22, 35, 43, 44, 64, 70, 75, 88, 90, 97, 110, 117
depth, vii, viii, 2, 102
determinants, iv, vii, viii, 11, 26, 35, 36, 40, 46, 55, 68, 75, 76, 77, 84, 85, 86, 89, 90, 91, 94
diabetes, 5, 7, 8, 9, 23, 27, 30, 32, 33, 39, 40, 46, 51, 58
disability, 88, 102
discharge instructions, 12, 38
dissatisfaction, 9, 68, 86, 89, 113
drug treatment, 88, 97

E

eating disorders, 75, 90
education, 71, 112
emergency, 2, 6, 7, 12, 17, 23, 30, 69, 88
emergency department, 2, 6, 7, 11, 17, 27, 28, 29, 30, 31, 34, 35, 38, 40, 41, 42, 48, 50, 53, 54, 55, 56, 58, 60, 62, 64, 65
emergency medicine, 23, 27, 28, 29, 32, 35, 36, 41, 50, 54, 55, 58, 62, 64
emergency physician, 12
emotion regulation, 82, 87
empathy, 71, 76, 78
environment, 4, 69, 76, 81, 87, 91

environment/organization of the service, 76
evidence, vii, viii, 2, 3, 9, 12, 16, 19, 23, 24, 70, 89, 94
expectations, viii, ix, 2, 16, 47, 48, 68, 76, 79, 87, 90, 91, 100, 101, 113, 119
experience, vii, 1, 2, 3, 4, 7, 8, 9, 11, 12, 13, 20, 22, 24, 25, 27, 29, 36, 42, 43, 48, 62, 63, 72, 74, 79, 81, 85, 92, 95
externalizing disorders, 84

F

factor analysis, 71
families, vii, viii, 1, 67, 69, 78, 80, 91
family therapy, 90, 94
feelings, 76, 81, 82, 87, 91
fibromyalgia, 23, 25, 41, 59
fracture, 16, 29, 40, 42
functional status, 11, 16, 17

G

gastroenterology, 21, 27, 37, 46, 55, 65
general practitioner, 29
general surgery, 14
glycosylated hemoglobin, 8
group therapy, 69
guideline, 8, 9, 11, 13, 21
gynecology, 18

H

HCAHPS, 2, 3, 10, 11, 24, 31, 32, 40, 41, 45, 53, 59, 60, 62
headache, 20, 27
health, ix, 2, 6, 7, 8, 9, 11, 12, 14, 18, 19, 20, 23, 24, 56, 61, 68, 71, 89, 97, 100, 101, 102, 114, 117
health care, 2, 6, 12, 20, 23
health care cost, 23, 59
health care costs, 23
health care system, 2
health care utilization, 6, 20
health outcomes, 9, 18, 23, 24, 31, 32, 37, 45, 53, 61
health status, 7, 14, 19, 20, 23, 45, 56, 61, 65
healthcare quality, 3, 27, 34, 39, 95
healthcare utilization, 6, 7, 21
heart disease, 6, 11, 21
heart failure, 7, 10, 11, 21, 35, 42, 60
hip fractures, 13
hip replacement, 16
history, 80, 84, 89, 100
hospitalization, viii, 1, 5, 69, 93

I

implants, 100, 109, 113, 116, 117, 118
improvements, viii, 67, 69
incidence, 101, 104, 111
individual character, viii, 68, 76, 91
individual characteristics, viii, 68, 76, 91
infection, 9, 17
inflammatory bowel disease, 21
injury, iv, 40
inpatient, viii, 2, 4, 6, 10, 11, 12, 17, 20, 21, 22, 23, 29, 38, 41, 44, 48, 62, 68, 69, 70, 71, 74, 75, 76, 80, 81, 82, 84, 85, 86, 87, 88, 90, 93, 95, 96, 97
Institute of Medicine, 2, 42
integration, viii, 67, 70
intensive care unit, 13
inter-individual variables, 76, 85, 91
intervention, 7, 22, 70, 72, 77, 113
intra-individual characteristics, viii, 68, 76, 84, 91
invasive cancer, 115
issues, 3, 4, 6, 8, 12, 79, 86

J

joint replacement, 17, 40

K

knee-replacement, 17

L

length of stay, 13, 14, 17, 18, 33, 42, 60, 64
likelihood to recommend, 10, 19
limitations, 10, 20, 24, 101
liver cancer, 20
liver disease, 22
lower respiratory tract infection, 9
lung cancer, 14, 19
lupus, 23, 28, 35, 43, 61, 63

M

malpractice, 6, 46, 56
marital status, 112
mastectomy, viii, 99, 100, 103, 104, 105, 108, 109, 112, 113, 114, 115, 117, 118
measurement, ix, 3, 22, 24, 63, 93, 100, 101
medical, vii, 1, 6, 12, 19, 23, 78, 87, 106, 109
medical errors, 6
medication, viii, 1, 4, 5, 9, 12, 20, 22, 23, 51, 84, 88, 89
medication adherence, viii, 1, 4, 5, 9, 12, 20, 22, 23, 26, 27, 45, 51, 58
medicine, 23, 30, 68, 96
mental disorder, 69, 97
mental health, 68, 69, 70, 71, 74, 75, 77, 80, 83, 92, 94, 95, 96, 97, 102
mental health professionals, 71
meta-analysis, 5, 115
morbidity, 100, 101, 103, 104, 107, 108

mortality, viii, 2, 3, 4, 5, 9, 10, 11, 12, 13, 14, 16, 18, 19, 20, 21, 23, 30, 38, 42, 43, 47, 49, 55, 56, 60, 62
motivation, 70, 80, 90
multidimensional, 95
multiple informants, 68
multiple perspectives, v, viii, 67, 70, 88, 97
myocardial infarction, 10, 11, 13, 21, 34, 38, 49, 55, 58

N

neurology, 20, 64
neurosurgery, 17, 35, 41, 44, 53, 56, 60
nosocomial infections, 10, 13

O

obesity, 118
obstetrics, 18
online, 8, 10, 14, 36, 45, 47, 113, 114, 115, 116, 117, 118, 119
online ratings, 8, 10, 36
opioid, 8, 16, 29, 31, 36, 37, 38, 42, 46, 48, 51, 52, 60
opioids, 9, 10, 16, 18, 59
orthopedic, 16, 34, 53
outcomes, iv, v, vii, ix, 1, 3, 4, 8, 9, 10, 11, 12, 13, 17, 18, 19, 20, 21, 22, 23, 24, 26, 28, 29, 30, 32, 33, 35, 38, 39, 43, 44, 45, 46, 47, 49, 51, 52, 53, 54, 55, 57, 58, 59, 61, 65, 74, 93, 100, 101, 102, 103, 104, 107, 109, 110, 111, 112, 114, 115, 116, 117, 118, 119
outpatient, viii, 1, 2, 3, 9, 10, 20, 22, 23, 37, 44, 57, 69, 71, 72, 74, 75, 77, 93, 94, 95, 97
outpatient care, 2, 4, 22, 57, 71
over-testing, 9, 12, 23
over-treatment, 12, 23

P

pain, 8, 9, 12, 13, 14, 15, 16, 17, 18, 21, 22, 24, 27, 28, 29, 35, 38, 40, 41, 42, 46, 49, 50, 51, 53, 54, 55, 59, 102
pancreatic cancer, 19
parents, viii, 67, 69, 70, 74, 75, 76, 78, 81, 82, 83, 84, 85, 86, 87, 88, 89, 90, 91, 93, 94, 95, 96, 97
patient centered, 6, 7, 11
patient experience, iv, v, vii, 1, 2, 3, 4, 5, 6, 8, 9, 11, 12, 13, 14, 15, 18, 19, 20, 23, 24, 25, 26, 27, 32, 33, 34, 35, 37, 38, 39, 40, 43, 47, 48, 52, 59, 60, 62
patient reported outcomes, ix, 17, 100, 101, 102, 103, 107, 109
patient safety, 14, 60
patient satisfaction, iv, v, vii, ix, 1, 2, 3, 4, 5, 7, 8, 9, 10, 11, 12, 13, 14, 15, 18, 19, 20, 21, 22, 23, 25, 26, 27, 28, 29, 30, 31, 32, 33, 34, 35, 36, 38, 39, 40, 41, 42, 43, 44, 45, 46, 47, 48, 49, 51, 52, 53, 55, 56, 57, 58, 59, 61, 62, 63, 64, 65, 92, 93, 95, 99, 100, 102, 103, 106, 108, 110, 111, 112, 113, 116, 117, 118, 119
pelvic inflammatory disease, 12
peptic ulcer disease, 21
personalized medicine, 68
physical well-being, 105, 107, 109, 111
physicians, vii, 1, 4, 5, 6, 8, 16, 19, 22
plastic surgery, 15, 45, 99, 108, 114, 115
pneumonia, 10, 13, 37, 54
postoperative nausea and vomiting, 15
Press-Ganey, 2, 11, 17
primary care, 3, 4, 6, 7, 8, 9, 20, 25, 30, 31, 34, 38, 39, 40, 44, 46, 48, 50, 51, 52, 53, 56, 57, 62, 63, 64, 65
professionals, 23, 69, 76, 78, 90, 97
prognosis, 19, 76, 87
prophylactic, 103, 114
prostate cancer, 19
prosthesis, ix, 100
psoriasis, 21, 44, 56, 62
psychiatric diagnosis, 70
psychiatry, 22, 37, 38, 44, 61, 64, 65, 67, 92, 93, 94, 96, 97
psychopathology, 75, 80, 84, 89
psychosocial functioning, 109
psychosocial support, 110
psychotherapy, 69, 94
public health, 69

Q

QoL, 7, 11, 18, 20, 21, 22, 23, 102, 107
quality, iv, v, vii, ix, 2, 3, 5, 6, 7, 8, 9, 10, 11, 12, 13, 14, 15, 17, 18, 19, 21, 22, 23, 24, 26, 27, 28, 29, 30, 31, 32, 33, 34, 35, 36, 38, 39, 40, 42, 43, 44, 45, 46, 47, 48, 49, 51, 52, 53, 54, 56, 57, 58, 59, 60, 61, 62, 63, 64, 65, 76, 78, 79, 80, 85, 94, 95, 99, 100, 102, 103, 105, 106, 107, 110, 111, 112, 113, 114, 115, 116, 117, 118, 119
quality measures, 8, 10, 11, 13, 14, 35, 43, 62
quality of life, iv, vii, ix, 7, 24, 26, 35, 44, 47, 51, 52, 64, 79, 80, 95, 99, 100, 102, 103, 105, 106, 107, 110, 111, 112, 114, 116, 117, 118, 119
quality of service, 12
questionnaire, ix, 29, 71, 72, 74, 100, 101, 102, 108, 110, 114

R

radiation, viii, 99, 100, 105, 106
readmission, 7, 14, 17, 29, 37, 42, 59
reconstruction, vii, ix, 99, 100, 101, 102, 103, 104, 105, 106, 107, 108, 109, 110, 111, 112, 113, 114, 115, 116, 117, 118, 119

recovery, 15, 101, 108
recruiting, 105, 107
recurrence, 104, 115
regression analysis, 109
reimbursement, vii, 1, 3, 10, 13, 24
relationship, 4, 5, 6, 9, 14, 17, 19, 20, 26, 27, 29, 35, 38, 39, 40, 42, 43, 44, 45, 46, 47, 51, 57, 60, 61, 71, 76, 78, 79, 80, 82, 83, 85, 86, 91, 94, 96
retrospective, 6, 7, 8, 10, 19, 20, 24, 41, 94, 110
revenue, 4, 13
rheumatoid arthritis, 23, 28
rheumatology, 22, 25, 29, 43, 61
risk, 4, 6, 11, 16, 104, 110, 113, 115

S

satisfaction, iv, v, vii, viii, 1, 2, 3, 4, 6, 7, 8, 9, 10, 11, 12, 13, 14, 15, 16, 17, 18, 19, 20, 21, 22, 23, 24, 25, 26, 28, 29, 34, 37, 40, 41, 42, 43, 44, 45, 48, 49, 51, 52, 53, 55, 56, 57, 59, 60, 64, 65, 67, 68, 69, 70, 71, 72, 74, 75, 76, 77, 78, 79, 80, 81, 82, 83, 84, 85, 86, 87, 88, 89, 90, 91, 92, 93, 94, 95, 96, 97, 100, 102, 103, 104, 107, 108, 110, 111, 112, 113, 117
schizophrenia, 22, 37, 44, 76, 84, 93
self-esteem, 100, 109
self-expression, 81
self-image, 110
self-reported health, 7
services, iv, viii, 4, 52, 68, 69, 71, 72, 74, 80, 82, 87, 92, 94
shoulder surgery, 16
side effects, 19, 22, 23, 81, 102
spine surgery, 17, 41, 46, 48, 49, 50, 60
stroke, 5, 7, 13, 20, 26, 32, 55, 60, 65
substance abuse, 75, 79
substance use, 90

surgery, ix, 10, 14, 15, 16, 17, 18, 28, 29, 32, 34, 35, 39, 40, 42, 43, 45, 47, 49, 50, 51, 52, 53, 57, 59, 61, 62, 63, 100, 101, 103, 105, 109, 112, 113, 114, 115, 116, 117, 118
surgical care, 13, 18, 23, 47, 62
surgical intervention, 112
surrogate outcome, 5, 8, 9, 34
survival, viii, 19, 99
survival rate, viii, 99
survivors, viii, 20, 99, 100, 114
symptoms, 7, 11, 14, 15, 17, 18, 21, 22, 23, 74, 80, 86, 102, 110, 117

T

target population, 101
testing, 9, 12, 21, 23, 102
therapeutic alliance, 22, 37, 78, 83, 85, 92
therapeutic process, 85
therapeutic relationship (or alliance), 90
therapist, 70, 76, 78, 80, 82, 85, 86, 88, 89, 90, 91, 97
therapy, 20, 82, 83, 88, 89, 95, 96, 102, 105, 106, 111, 113, 115
thoracic surgery, 14, 30, 59
thoughts, 70, 76, 82
trauma, 16, 26, 28, 32, 33, 35, 43, 56, 62, 64
treatment, viii, 9, 12, 18, 19, 21, 23, 44, 67, 69, 70, 71, 72, 73, 76, 77, 78, 79, 80, 81, 82, 83, 84, 85, 86, 87, 88, 89, 90, 91, 93, 94, 95, 96, 97, 99, 102, 104, 105, 106, 108, 117
treatment outcomes, viii, 68, 76, 86, 91
trial, 7, 8, 9, 107, 108

U

ulcers, 10
urology, 18
utilization, 6, 51

V

vaccination, 5
validation, 95, 101
variables, ix, 24, 76, 77, 91, 94, 96, 100, 110, 113
vascular surgery, 14, 53
venous thromboembolism, 10

W

wait times, 4, 12, 23, 30, 55
well-being, 103, 105, 107, 109, 111
worldwide, viii, 99, 100

Y

young people, 90, 97
young women, 101